Understanding Mental Health Practice

Sara Miller McCune founded SAGE Publishing in 1965 to support the dissemination of usable knowledge and educate a global community. SAGE publishes more than 1000 journals and over 800 new books each year, spanning a wide range of subject areas. Our growing selection of library products includes archives, data, case studies and video. SAGE remains majority owned by our founder and after her lifetime will become owned by a charitable trust that secures the company's continued independence.

Los Angeles | London | New Delhi | Singapore | Washington DC | Melbourne

Understanding Mental Health Practice

Mark Haith

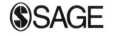

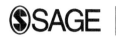

Learning Matters
An imprint of SAGE Publications Ltd
1 Oliver's Yard
55 City Road
London EC1Y 1SP

SAGE Publications Inc.
2455 Teller Road
Thousand Oaks, California 91320

SAGE Publications India Pvt Ltd
B 1/I 1 Mohan Cooperative Industrial Area
Mathura Road
New Delhi 110 044

SAGE Publications Asia-Pacific Pte Ltd
3 Church Street
#10-04 Samsung Hub
Singapore 049483

Editor: Alex Clabburn
Development editor: Eleanor Rivers
Production controller: Chris Marke
Project management: Swales & Willis Ltd,
Exeter, Devon
Marketing manager: Camille Richmond
Cover design: Wendy Scott
Typeset by: C&M Digitals (P) Ltd, Chennai, India
Printed in the UK

First published 2018

Library of Congress Control Number: 2017954830

British Library Cataloguing in Publication data

A catalogue record for this book is available from
the British Library

ISBN: 978-1-4739-6653-6
ISBN: 978-1-4739-6654-3 (pbk)

Contents

Transforming Nursing Practice is a series tailor-made for pre-registration student nurses. Each book in the series is:

- Affordable
- Mapped to the NMC Standards and Essential Skills Clusters
- Full of active learning features
- Focused on applying theory to practice

Each book addresses a core topic and they have been carefully developed to be simple to use, quick to read and written in clear language.

> An invaluable series of books that explicitly relates to the NMC standards. Each book cover a different topic that students need to explore in order to develop into a qualified nurse... I would recommend this series to all Pre-Registration nursing students whatever their field or year of study
>
> **Linda Robson**
> **Senior Lecturer, Edge Hill University**
>
> The set of books is an excellent resource for students. The series is small, easily portable and valuable. I use the whole set on a regular basis.
>
> **Fiona Davies**
> **Senior Nurse Lecturer, University of Derby**
>
> I recommend the SAGE/Learning Matters series to all my students as they are relevant and concise. Please keep up the good work.
>
> **Thomas Beary**
> **Senior Lecturer in Mental Health Nursing, University of Hertfordshire**

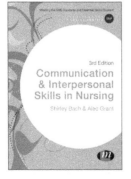

3rd Edition
Communication & Interpersonal Skills in Nursing
Shirley Bach & Alec Grant

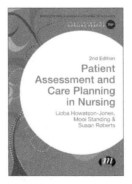

2nd Edition
Patient Assessment and Care Planning in Nursing
Lioba Howatson-Jones, Mooi Standing & Susan Roberts

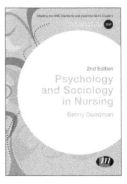

2nd Edition
Psychology and Sociology in Nursing
Benny Goodman

You can find more information on each of these titles and our other learning resources at www.sagepub.co.uk. Many of these titles are also available in various e-book formats, please visit our website for more information.

About the author

Mark Haith is Senior Lecturer in Mental Health, Isle of Man. He was previously a Lecturer in Mental Health at the Universities of Kent, West of England, Robert Gordon and Abertay. He has also worked as a community mental health nurse in Child and Adolescent Mental Health services in Canterbury.

Acknowledgements

I couldn't have written this book without the help of Test Match Special and a belief in myself.

The publisher would like to thank Dr Sandra Walker for her valuable feedback during the development process and continued support as Mental Health series editor for the Transforming Nursing Practice series. We would also like to thank Diane Wills for her input and ideas when the book was initially being conceptualised.

Dedication

For our patients and for our students – change will only come if you make it.

Alle meravigliose persone della comunità terapeutica "San Patrignano". Vorrei tanto trovarmi li, perchè il *Vostro* è davvero il miglior modo di vivere.

Al Sig. Sergio. Questo libro lo dedico a te, come richiesto. Un giorno avrò anche io un *"Olympo"*. Prima di allora, sicuramente torneremo a trovarvi. *Claudio Buon anno nuovo!*

For Karen, Sarah, Yusuf and Raymond for believing in me.

For Mum and Dad, for your love and support.

For Verity and Boudica, for never doubting that I would achieve it. I love you both. Xxx.

..02000.0000000..20000....23022.
3.663030000.122222220

.3..

63

Introduction

Who is this book for?

This book is written with a particular focus for mental health nursing students. It also has scope to be of interest to qualified health professionals wishing to improve their understanding of mental health and wellbeing. For this reason, it may be particularly useful for nurses and other health professionals who do not work for mental health services, but recognise the impact of mental health factors within their own work.

Why *Understanding Mental Health Practice*?

Mental health is commonly overlooked by both specialist and general health service providers. It is a term that is often misused in discussions of psychological and behavioural difficulties. This is not surprising when we recognise that the National Health Service is in reality a national illness service. Within professional training courses, the main focus remains on understanding causes and presentations of mental illness. Experiences from working with pre-registration students suggest that their overwhelming interest when beginning mental health nurse education is on understanding mental illness. This situation is also apparent in mental health practice, as very few genuine mental health services exist in the public sector. When asked about psychiatric and mental health nursing, few students or practitioners recognise any difference between these terms, using them interchangeably. Mental illness and mental health are inter-related but separate concepts; without promoting an understanding of mental health for students and qualified health professionals this misunderstanding will continue. Recognising mental health as a central factor for physical and psychological wellbeing is necessary to provide effective future services across all areas of healthcare.

Book structure

Chapter 1 focuses on mental and physical health and wellbeing. It challenges the assumption that they are separate aspects of the person, instead proposing them as intrinsically interlinked factors. Physical and mental health issues can be seen to cause each other, so it is argued that effective treatment must address both aspects of personal wellbeing simultaneously.

Chapter 2 examines a range of common mental health conditions proposed by the ICD-10 and DSM-5 statistical manuals. Through appreciating the symptoms required for a diagnosis to be made, the reader is equipped with an ability to question their value in practice. This creates an informed viewpoint useful for a student or health professional advocating for a patient when a disputable diagnosis has been given.

Chapter 3 considers suicide risk in mental healthcare. It examines the links and differences between suicide and self-harm. Suicide risk factors are discussed, and the limitations of suicide assessment processes are recognised. As a result, an individualised approach to working with people at potential risk of suicide is proposed. The powers provided by commonly used sections of the Mental Health Act (1983) are examined to explain the role of this legislation in keeping people who are at risk of suicide safe.

Chapter 4 examines mental health assessment and care planning. It considers the nursing assessment process, looking in detail at the Roper, Logan and Tierney activities of living model as a holistic assessment of need. This is not a mental health specific approach, but it is particularly useful because it covers a much broader range of inter-related physical and psychological health issues impacting on mental wellbeing.

Chapter 5 considers four of the major psychotherapeutic approaches to mental healthcare. Developing a working knowledge of these approaches allows us to explain to our patients how specialist therapeutic treatment works, as well as determining what information is most relevant when making referrals for treatment. Knowledge of these psychotherapeutic approaches is critical for our effective care of the patient, as it allows the practitioner to recognise and challenge unhealthy behaviour and thinking patterns.

Chapter 6 concerns drug treatments for mental health issues. Each medicine is considered in terms of the conditions it is used to treat, as well as pre-existing conditions that prohibit its use. Side-effects are explained for each drug as a means of helping care staff to provide this information for their patients. This allows service users an informed choice regarding their use, something that is under-provided in mental health practice.

Chapter 7 examines recovery from mental health problems. This includes an understanding of the philosophy of recovery-based approaches, and techniques used to achieve recovery in practice. The clash between recovery and psychiatric practice highlights the need for a revolutionary change in the aims and methods of modern mental health services.

Requirements for the *NMC Standards for Pre-registration Nursing Education* and the *Essential Skills Clusters*

The Nursing and Midwifery Council (NMC) has established standards of competence to be met by applicants to different parts of the register, and these are the standards it considers necessary for safe and effective practice. In addition to the competencies, the NMC has set out specific skills that nursing students must be able to perform at various points of an education programme. These are known as Essential Skills Clusters (ESCs). This book is structured so that it will help you to understand and meet the competencies and ESCs required for entry to the NMC register. The relevant competencies and ESCs are presented at the start of each chapter so that you can clearly see which ones the chapter addresses. There are *generic standards* that all nursing students irrespective of their field must achieve, and *field-specific standards* relating to each field of nursing; i.e. mental health, children's, learning disability and adult nursing. All chapters have generic standards, and most also have field-specific standards listed as well.

This book includes the latest standards for 2010 onwards, taken from the *Standards for Pre-registration Nursing Education* (NMC, 2010).

Learning features

Learning from reading text is not always easy. Therefore, to provide variety and to assist with the development of independent learning skills and the application of theory to practice, this book contains activities, case studies, further reading, useful websites and other materials to enable you to participate in your own learning. You will need to develop your own study skills and "learn how to learn" to get the best from the material. The book cannot provide all the answers – but instead provides a framework for your learning.

The activities in the book will in particular help you to make sense of, and learn about, the material being presented. Some activities ask you to reflect on aspects of practice, or your experience of it, or the people or situations you encounter. *Reflection* is an essential skill in nursing, and it helps you to understand the world around you and often to identify how things might be improved. Other activities will help you develop key graduate skills such as your ability to *think critically* about a topic in order to challenge received wisdom. Communication and working as part of a team are core to all nursing practice, and some activities will ask you to think about your *communication skills* to help develop these. Finally, as a registered nurse you will be expected to *lead and manage* your own team, case load or area of care, and so some activities focus on helping you build confidence in doing this.

All the activities require you to take a break from reading the text, think through the issues presented and carry out some independent study, possibly using the internet. Where appropriate, there are sample answers presented at the end of each chapter, and these will help you to understand more fully your own reflections and independent study. Remember, academic study will always require independent work; attending lectures will never be enough to be successful on your programme, and these activities will help to deepen your knowledge and understanding of the issues under scrutiny and give you practice at working on your own.

You might want to think about completing these activities as part of your personal development plan (PDP) or portfolio. After completing the activity write it up in your PDP or portfolio in a section devoted to that particular skill, then look back over time to see how far you are developing. You can also do more of the activities for a key skill that you have identified a weakness in, which will help build your skill and confidence in this area.

This book also contains a glossary on page 154 to assist you with unfamiliar terms. Glossary terms are in bold in the first instance that they appear.

Chapter 1
Mental and physical health and wellbeing

NMC Standards for Pre-registration Nursing Education

This chapter will address the following competencies:

Domain 1: Professional values

3.1   Mental health nurses must promote mental health and wellbeing, while challenging the inequalities and discrimination that may arise from or contribute to mental health problems.

Domain 3: Nursing practice and decision-making

8.1   Mental health nurses must practise in a way that promotes the self-determination and expertise of people with mental health problems, using a range of approaches and tools that aid wellness and recovery and enable self-care and self-management.

NMC Essential Skills Clusters

This chapter will address the following ESC:

Cluster: Organisational aspects of care

9.16 Promotes health and wellbeing, self-care and independence by teaching and empowering people and carers to make choices in coping with the effects of treatment and the ongoing nature and likely consequences of a condition including death and dying.

Chapter aims

By the end of the chapter you will be able to:

- recognise factors indicating mental health;
- understand the falsity of assuming that "mental health" and "mental illness" are the same thing;
- describe the relationships between physical health and mental health, and between physical illness and mental illness.

Introduction

Case study: A poorly designed mental health unit

My first experiences of a mental health unit were shocking. This wasn't because of the types of patients that I met, or the nature of their conditions, but the environment within which they were treated. The ward consisted of a series of small rooms branching off a long corridor, making it dark and emphasising its cramped nature. Because the lines of sight were entirely restricted, some nursing staff patrolled the ward to ensure they knew where the patients were, and what they were doing. Other staff took a different approach, isolating themselves in the nursing office. The most striking thing about this treatment centre was the complete lack of consideration for stimulation provided for patients. Walls were plain without pictures or other decoration. There was a lack of organised activity for patients, resulting in the few events of the day gaining disproportionate significance. Beyond meals and drug rounds, patients spent their time smoking, drinking tea, eating junk food and sleeping. The atmosphere fluctuated from subdued to aggressive depending on how boredom affected the patient group at the time.

This case study depicts a mental health unit that is anything but healthy. Although the situation described occurred many years ago, and there are examples of much better approaches to inpatient mental healthcare, this type of unhealthy psychiatric setting remains far from exceptional. Advances in mental health treatment have been significant over recent years, in particular through the recognition of psychological therapies as a vital form of treatment, but physical wellbeing remains undervalued in mental health practice. Starting with the right physical environment is critical to providing treatment that is physically and mentally healthy.

Modern health services typically treat mental and physical health issues in isolation from each other. This is despite interlinking cause and effect widely recognised between them. Poor physical wellbeing is a major cause of mental ill health; therefore improving physical health is critical within effective mental health treatment (Sanna et al., 2013; Tansella et al., 2014).

This chapter highlights the importance of treating both aspects of health as one interlinked care package. It begins by exploring psychotherapeutic perspectives of mental health, then considers the predominance of mental illness within health services. The relationship between physical and mental illness is discussed, followed by physical and mental wellness. Through understanding the differences between these widely interchangeable terms, a more informed approach to mental and physical health is possible.

Defining mental health

An influential definition of mental health comes from the World Health Organization (WHO), suggesting it is:

... a state of wellbeing in which the individual realizes his or her own abilities, can cope with the normal stresses of life, can work productively and fruitfully, and is able to make a contribution to his or her community.

(WHO, 2001, p. 1)

Although it has some worth, there are a number of issues apparent with this definition, warranting further investigation. Fully realising our abilities is rare for any individual; where it occurs, it is transient rather than permanent. Mental health defined by these factors would therefore also be rare and transient, making it an unrealistically high standard. Conversely, an ability to "cope with the normal stresses of life" seems an unrealistically low standard. Not being able to deal with normal stresses may indicate mental illness, but coping with everyday occurrences seems insufficient to signify mental wellness. Productivity at work could occur in a mentally well person, but its absence does not exclude mental health. Not every person needs or desires to work; if we instead extend the term "work" to cover constructive activities, a more useful understanding emerges. The idea of contribution to community suggests that mental health occurs through successful social interaction; this is probably the case most, but not all, of the time.

The WHO definition contains both useful and disputable points. This suggests that we need to consider alternative views on mental health. Practical approaches to achieving **mental wellbeing** are provided by the major psychotherapeutic modalities. A consideration of psychodynamic theory, cognitive behaviour therapy, the person-centred approach, brief solution-focused therapy and mindfulness approaches may provide a more helpful understanding of mental health than the WHO definition alone. As we will see, a lack of consensus exists within psychotherapeutic approaches regarding a definition of mental health.

Psychotherapeutic perspectives of mental health

The original purpose of psychotherapy was to reduce symptoms of mental illness. Modern approaches also address improvement of mental wellbeing in people without psychiatric symptoms. Psychodynamic theories remain highly influential in the diagnostic approach to psychiatry, defining specific mental illnesses through patients' symptoms. This is a long-term approach, sometimes lasting for years. Symptoms of mental illness are viewed as the result of psychological complexes occurring during childhood. Mental wellbeing is viewed as the absence of mental illness within psychodynamic therapies.

Cognitive behaviour therapy (CBT) provides more balanced views of mental illness and mental health. It proposes objective, free-thinking decision-making as the basis of healthy emotions and behaviour. Conversely, subjective rule-based decisions cause emotional distress and unhealthy behaviours. The presence of habitual unhelpful thinking is due to conditioned (automatic) responses resulting from traumatic experiences. From a CBT perspective, mental wellbeing occurs through becoming aware of personal conditioned responses and replacing them with decisions based on realistic evidence. The process of reconditioning our thoughts, feelings and behaviour using a CBT approach is described within the following case study.

Case study: An example of mental health work using CBT principles

Yaz Husain has been working on improving her self-esteem for the last fourteen weeks with Mike, a community mental health worker. She has gained a great deal of insight through the process, recognising the impact her negative thinking has on how she feels about herself and other people. Through identifying situations that cause her distress, she has been able to plan strategies that allow her to cope more effectively with her fears. She recognises her negative thought patterns are part of the reason friends and family members are able to take advantage of her good nature; in order to avoid potential confrontation, Yaz offers childcare even though she feels this is unfair on her. Discussing her thoughts, feelings and actions with Mike has allowed Yaz to plan a new way of reacting to childcare requests, which is to politely refuse except in cases of emergency. Yaz recognises that early experiences of rejection have been highly influential in encouraging her to do what family members want in case they reject her again. By changing her actions, Yaz now appreciates that relationships do not end if she doesn't put other people's needs ahead of her own. As a result of this new understanding, she feels that her own mental health has improved.

The work undertaken by Yaz is an example of a mental health intervention creating behavioural change that influences her wider experience of life. Activity 1.1 asks you to consider aspects of your own conditioning.

Activity 1.1   *Reflection*

Consider the work Yaz has been undertaking using principles of CBT. Are there any areas of your own life where previous experiences encourage you to act in a manner that you don't feel comfortable with?

Because this is a personal piece of reflection, a suggested answer is not available at the end of the chapter.

Recognising the influence of previous experiences on our actions allows us to appreciate the potential benefit of CBT on mental wellbeing. Where CBT seeks to develop a pattern of cause and effect between thoughts, emotions and behaviour, brief solution-focused therapy (BSFT) takes a simpler approach to behaviour change. It seeks to change perspective from focusing on the impact of a problem, to considering how solutions can realistically be achieved. Through encouraging action to make necessary changes, troubling situations become opportunities to achieve difficult challenges. Self-belief replaces self-doubt once the person has developed positive problem-solving skills. BSFT therefore demonstrates that good mental health requires an ability to achieve solutions for the difficulties we experience. Clay's case study illustrates the use of BSFT principles in action.

Case study: Using principles from brief solution-focused therapy to improve difficult situations

Clay has been unemployed for the last two years following more than 20 years in a senior industrial role. He is bitter about the means of his dismissal which he believes wasn't through any fault of his own. He has been using his savings to maintain his lifestyle and is close to running out of money. He has been interviewed regularly for a number of promising jobs, but has repeatedly failed to be offered employment. He is concerned that he may have been "blacklisted" within the industry, and the anxiety he is experiencing to get a job is reducing his performance. His family are unaware of his present circumstances and he tends to avoid former colleagues, so has become isolated from other people. He feels that his mental health is the poorest it has been for a long time.

Due to his business background, Clay is aware of solution-focused approaches to challenging situations. Following his latest rejection for employment, he formally evaluates his options. By putting aside his bitterness towards his situation, Clay recognises that he remains attractive to the right employer, but that he has not yet found them. He also knows that even multiple rejections do not justify his fears that he is worthless as a person or employee. The options Clay identifies are: to continue applying for work within his own industry; to seek this type of work elsewhere; or to look at different jobs entirely. Clay decides to have one last try for a promising job elsewhere in the country before trying something entirely different. The match between himself and the employer is great and he is offered the job. After three years in post Clay feels this is the best job he has had in many years; he is settled and financially more successful than before, with prospects of further promotion. He can see that the problem with gaining employment did not come from him, but sits with the companies he applied to, who seem to value a less experienced and cheaper employee above an experienced person like himself. Clay feels mentally well and more compassionate for others undergoing workplace difficulties of this kind.

BSFT allows Clay to re-evaluate his approach to work and his life. Following his example, Activity 1.2 asks you to refocus on solutions for difficult situations within your own life.

Activity 1.2   *Reflection*

Consider a recent situation where you felt out of control. Concentrate on switching your thoughts from the emotional impact that the situation has on you, to considering what you can do personally to resolve the issue.

Is any sort of positive progress possible in your situation, and if so, how does this realisation affect you emotionally?

Because this is a personal piece of reflection, a suggested answer is not available at the end of the chapter.

Having considered Clay's example and your own reflections, we can now examine the person-centred approach (PCA) to personal development. Clay's example demonstrates BSFT in facilitating a change of focus from problem to solution. PCA shares BSFT's emphasis on self-reliance, but provides a more developed theory of mental wellbeing. Accepting self-responsibility for poor mental health also means accepting personal ability to make changes to improve matters. Mental health is therefore achievable through individuals making the choices required to ascertain what they personally need. The PCA assists the individual to move from an **incongruent** (dishonest) way of being, to **congruence** in their thoughts, feelings and behaviour. Harmony between these factors enables the person to be mentally well. Conversely, a person avoiding expression of their real thoughts, feelings or behaviour is likely to experience psychological disturbance. The PCA suggests decision-making free from external influence, creativity and honest self-expression only occurs through personal congruence. The degree of congruence experienced by the individual is seen in the PCA as determining their mental health. An illustration of the development of personal congruence is given in the next case study.

Case study: Developing congruence using the person-centred approach

Juan began counselling using the person-centred approach after many years of unsuccessful treatment for depression using antidepressants. Through building a trusting relationship with Alan, a mental health professional with experience in counselling, Juan has been able to verbalise his feelings in an increasingly honest and clear manner. Alan's role is not to advise Juan, but instead to accept his thoughts, feelings and behaviour without judgement. Over a number of weeks Juan was able to explain to Alan his regrets at being unable to express his sexuality freely because he fears upsetting his wife. Juan sees living separately as the only realistic way of being himself. However, he does not feel he has the right to divorce his wife because of the upset this will cause his family, who he loves very much. He has remained stuck in this way of thinking until breaking down in front of his wife and telling her openly about his feelings. Although difficult for her, she has accepted the reality of the situation. They have agreed to live apart but with regular contact for the sake of the whole family. Juan feels revealing his feelings has allowed him to be fully himself for the first time. He is much happier about himself and his life. As he is no longer experiencing symptoms of depression, he has reduced his antidepressant use with a view to being drug-free in the longer term.

The mental health work undertaken by Juan demonstrates the self-reflective nature of the PCA. To encourage congruence within other people, mental health professionals need to become as congruent as possible themselves. The question therefore arising at this point is: how congruent are you in your own life? Activity 1.3 looks at this question further.

Activity 1.3   *Reflection*

Consider the things you would most like to do with your life. To what extent do you hold back from doing them because of fears that other people will judge you negatively?

Because this is a personal piece of reflection, a suggested answer is not available at the end of the chapter.

Having considered the experiences of Juan and undertaken a personal assessment of your own congruence, the challenging nature of the PCA becomes apparent. The self-reflective aspect of PCA shares much with mindfulness-based approaches. Theories of **mindfulness** suggest that becoming non-judgemental towards others allows us to become less critical of ourselves. Acceptance of reality, through recognition of the things we can change and those that we cannot, is a view of mental wellbeing proposed within mindfulness. This recognition of possibilities is used to guide our actions in achieving what is realistic for ourselves. Determination is required to accept self-responsibility for personal wellbeing, as we naturally tend to blame other people and external events for our unhappiness. Mindfulness suggests the ability to flexibly meet the needs of each individual situation as it occurs, and determine emotional wellbeing. By focusing on the reality of the present, we are able to recognise and therefore let go of unrealistic expectations felt towards other people, and excessive **attachment** to material objects. In the next case study, we see Judit using mindfulness to improve her mental health.

Case study: Mindfulness practice for a more fulfilling life

Following a divorce as a young woman, Judit has concentrated on being successful in her career. She values financial independence and business standing rather than personal relationships within her life. She prefers her own company, but does like time with certain other people. Although she enjoys her life, things still feel incomplete for her. Sometimes she feels lonely and depressed without understanding why. Judit does not want to address these issues through therapy or taking antidepressants, but sees the value in becoming more aware of what is happening for her through mindfulness. Over a period of time, Judit practises becoming more focused on present situations. She recognises that she has more of a tendency to isolate herself than she realised, so is working on becoming more social with people she trusts. Through self-reflection, Judit has begun to address her feelings of emptiness by allowing others into her life in a more meaningful way.

Judit's experience is an example of using mindfulness principles in an individualised manner that works for her. Activity 1.4 provides an opportunity to consider how mindfulness may improve personal effectiveness in the reader's own life.

Activity 1.4   *Reflection*

Consider an aspect of your life where you feel awkward. Focus on what actually happens in this situation, rather than what you think will probably happen. How does this affect your view of events?

Because this is a personal piece of reflection, a suggested answer is not available at the end of the chapter.

As can be appreciated through undertaking this mindfulness exercise, personal development through self-reflection is helpful for ongoing mental wellbeing.

Having reviewed a range of psychotherapeutic approaches towards mental health, we are presented with a number of useful ideas on the subject. These include identifying and reducing conditioned responses; honest expression of thoughts, feelings and behaviour; non-judgementalism towards self and others; developing an ability to focus on solutions rather than problems; and an acceptance of what we can and cannot change in guiding our actions. These factors highlight the need for professionals to develop an individualised approach to mental health work based on the needs of each service user. In comparison, a definition of mental health based on the absence of mental illness lacks sophistication necessary to usefully understand the complex needs of individuals. Unfortunately, this highly simplistic view predominates within most modern psychiatric systems.

The ongoing professional focus on mental illness rather than mental health

Traditionally, very few mental health nursing textbooks have addressed mental wellbeing, focusing instead on views of mental illness proposed by the DSM and ICD categorisation systems. This emphasis is revealed by a simple internet search. At the time of writing, over 325,000 search results were returned for the terms "psychiatric and mental health nursing" compared to only one for "psychiatric versus mental health nursing" (accurate as of January 2017). This suggests psychiatric and mental health nursing roles are not seen as distinct.

Because the terms "mental health" and "psychiatric" nurse are so widely interchangeable, it is useful to examine their meanings. Graduates are registered by the NMC as "Mental Health Nurses". This means "psychiatric nurse" is an obsolete term, despite being commonly used in practice. The role of a psychiatric nurse is seen by those using this title to be one of assisting in the provision of psychiatric care, a hierarchical system led by a psychiatrist. Psychiatric care has a major focus on public safety and the suppression of symptoms of mental illness through psychotropic medication. Mental health nursing represents a very different role, being concerned with the development of psychological wellbeing. This could be with a person who has never experienced symptoms of mental ill health, or it could be with a person who has substantial experience of symptoms. The nature of mental health work is expressive, individualised and unique to each individual, therefore the worker has far greater autonomy in their practice than is the case for a psychiatric nurse. A realistic balance needs to be created so that specialist services are able to provide both mental health and mental illness work for those in need. Disagreement among professionals regarding appropriate functions of mental health nurses includes their role regarding the physical health of patients with pre-existing mental health issues.

The relationship between physical and mental illness

Our examination of mental health must consider physical health. This is because mental and physical health issues commonly occur in the same individuals. Around a third of people experiencing long-term physical health issues also have mental health issues, and almost half of people whose main health concerns are psychological also experience chronic physical complaints. The relationship between **co-morbid** physical and mental health is **bidirectional** and complex (Sanna et al., 2013; Tansella et al., 2014). Poor appetite, sleep and lack of energy are common symptoms due to many physical health issues, but also occur as a result of mental illness (Laoutidis and Mathiak, 2013; Williams and Rajapakse, 2013). This makes diagnosing causes difficult and allows aspects of a person's ill health to be potentially missed.

Physical ill health may be depressing and cause anxiety. Mental health issues commonly impact on physical wellbeing, particularly through poor diet, lack of exercise and side-effects of medication (Amital et al., 2013). Physical and mental co-morbidity result in poorer **recovery** rates for people experiencing depression compared to depressed patients without physical health issues. It has been suggested that 5% of service users, represented by those with multiple co-morbid physical and mental health conditions, require around a third of health service budgets. This group predominantly live in socio-economically deprived areas, the experience of which is a major contributory factor for the emergence of mental health issues. People with severe mental illness are much more likely than the general population to be admitted to hospital for unplanned and preventable physical health treatments, and to remain longer once admitted (Payne et al., 2013; Sanna et al., 2013).

People diagnosed with depression are significantly more likely to experience heart conditions, dementia, diabetes, cancer, lung conditions, osteoarthritis and rheumatoid arthritis. These conditions represent the majority of long-term disability and mortality within developed nations. Symptoms and progress of these diseases, patients' ability to function, risk of complications and response to medication are significantly worse for anxious or depressed people (Sanna et al., 2013). After accounting for gender and age related factors, risk of death is more than double for people who experience significant anxiety, depression or alcoholism (Markkula et al., 2012).

Because people with severe mental health problems are much more likely to experience multiple health issues, they utilise services to a much higher degree than most consumers. Well-established trends in clinical practice should ensure that health services are designed to cater simultaneously for physical and mental health issues. Rather than recognising and acting on patient need through jointly coordinated and accessible services, a treatment gap between physical and mental healthcare exists. This is due to an inability by most services to comprehensively diagnose and treat patients experiencing a spectrum of physical and mental health needs. Despite recognition of need for integrated multi-disciplinary services, this is far from the norm in either physical or mental healthcare settings. For example, only around a third of cancer survivors seeking psychological treatment are able to access this service (Nakash et al., 2013). Treatment typically remains specialised in treating single specific areas of concern rather then reacting to the reality of patient need, which often includes a wide range of inter-related physical and psychological issues. This results in people with severe mental health problems, who represent some of the most vulnerable people in society, being unable to access appropriate services for their needs.

To summarise the relationship between physical and mental illness, it is clear that to be effective the role of specialist mental health services must include physical health, because of the severity of need and lack of services available to patients. The next section of this chapter highlights the necessity of mental health services targeting physical wellbeing as a means of improving mental health.

The relationship between physical and mental wellness

Lack of exercise, poor nutrition and sleep patterns occur in conjunction with many severe mental health problems, in particular for people experiencing anxiety, mood disorders or psychosis. Because of their prolific presence within the psychiatric population, there is no doubt that they need to be addressed as key issues for treatment by mental health professionals. These three factors are therefore of particular significance for discussion here.

Exercise may be viewed as both a treatment and a preventative factor for mental health issues (Sallis, 2009). Exercise increases the production of dopamine and serotonin in the brain, chemicals that psychotropic medicines seek to replace (see Chapter 6). Exercise is cost-effective, may be safely used in conjunction with other treatments, and lacks the side-effects that are so problematic in medicinal treatments of mental health issues (Fiuza-Luces et al., 2013).

The National Institute for Health and Care Excellence (NICE) recommends exercise as primary treatment for mild to moderate depression (NICE, 2010). Exercise lowers the risk of developing mood and anxiety disorders, regardless of age (Sjösten and Kivelä, 2006; Diamond and Lee, 2011). For those already experiencing mental health issues, exercise and effective nutrition significantly improve symptoms of anxiety, depression and aggression (Anita and Bhawna, 2015). Psychotic symptoms may benefit but are less likely to be helped by exercise than are symptoms of low mood (Gorczynski and Faulkner, 2010). However, exercise is probably more important for mental health patients than any other factor. Lack of exercise and poor diet, combined with weight gain (commonplace as a result of antipsychotic medication), reduce the life expectancy of people diagnosed with schizophrenia by up to 20 years (Saha et al., 2007). The relationship between exercise and mental health is bidirectional, meaning poor mental health reduces the likelihood of a person exercising, and lack of exercise reduces a person's mental health (De Moor et al., 2008).

The right amount, appropriate type, intensity, duration and minimum weekly frequency are yet to be established for exercise programmes seeking to improve mental health. Consequently, standard exercise guidelines of 30 minutes of daily moderate physical activity are recommended for good mental health (Gorczynski and Faulkner, 2010). The type of exercise chosen is less relevant than ensuring the participation of those involved. It is important to build up exercise levels realistically when working with people with severe mental health issues if they have been extremely inactive. This could involve relative minor amounts of exercise if it represents significant change for the individual (Alvarez-Jimenez and González-Blanch, 2010). By establishing daily activity routines and appropriate social support, the maintenance of physical activity and longer-term symptom reduction becomes much more likely. There is a tendency for people with mental health issues to become de-motivated, and special consideration should be given to this (Wolff et al., 2011). Conversely, the ability of a mental health service user-led group to motivate members to remain active is extremely powerful, as this case study demonstrates.

Case study: Exercise as a prescription for mental health

*Jessie has long-term issues with maintaining a healthy weight, which have been worsened during the last six months by the use of **psychotropic medication**. She exercises irregularly and wishes to do more, but has always struggled with motivation due to embarrassment about her body shape. Jessie enrolled into an informal, gentle exercise class for people with mental health issues 8 weeks ago and has found this the most encouraging way to keep fit. The non-competitive nature of the group, and knowledge that all members either have their own mental health issues or are professionals with an interest in helping people with mental health problems has been extremely helpful for Jessie in maintaining regular attendance. She finds group activities helpful in ensuring that she is regularly active, but also in encouraging her to meet new people and to spend time away from her flat. Her sleep pattern has improved, and she feels less anxious. Jessie is working towards losing more weight in a controlled fashion through following the dietary advice of other members of the exercise group.*

Having considered a major lifestyle change made by Jessie to improve her mental health, Activity 1.5 reviews lifestyle factors that could be improved within your own life.

Activity 1.5   *Reflection*

Consider your own lifestyle. What simple improvements could you make in terms of your diet, the amount and quality of exercise you undertake, and the sleep you allow yourself?

Because this is a personal piece of reflection, a suggested answer is not available at the end of the chapter.

Jessie's example and your own reflections highlight the importance of physical health factors in maintaining good mental health. Having considered the impact of exercise on mental health, we should now consider the impact of diet on mental wellbeing. A healthy diet contains high amounts of vegetables, fruit, whole grains, fish, poultry and lower-fat dairy products (National Health and Medical Research Council, 2013). People eating this diet have higher life expectancy and lower prevalence of chronic health conditions (Scarborough et al., 2012; Wirt and Collins, 2009). A healthy diet also benefits emotional and cognitive wellbeing, so is therefore good for mental health (Kiecolt-Glaser, 2010). This is not the case for a typical unhealthy "Western" diet high in sugar, fat, snacks, processed meat and refined grains (Lai et al., 2014).

A healthy diet is associated with a reduced incidence of depression (Lai et al., 2014). Depressed people commonly use high-fat and high-sugar food in an attempt to alleviate anxiety or low mood. There appears to be a bidirectional relationship between depression and poor diet, both increasing the likelihood of the other (Christensen, 2001; Wurtman and Wurtman, 1989). Conversely, people who maintain a healthy diet are more likely to be physically active, nonsmokers, and use alcohol sensibly (Kourlaba et al., 2009; Whichelow and Prevost, 1996).

Exercise and diet are factors vital both to maintain mental health and prevent mental deterioration. A third equally important but often overlooked factor is sleep. There is a strong link between sleep disturbances, anxiety and depression across all age groups. Sleep issues with physical causes include narcolepsy, insomnia, **circadian rhythm disorders** and obstructive **sleep apnoea** (Spoormaker and Van Den Bout, 2005; Taylor et al., 2005). Other preventable factors negatively influencing sleep patterns include the influence of alcohol and drugs (including caffeine), the sleeper's environment, and excessive exercise or physical passivity (Alvaro et al., 2013).

A bidirectional relationship exists between a lack of quality sleep, and the prevalence of depression and anxiety symptoms. This suggests that these factors are both causes and consequences of each other (Jansson-Frojmark and Lindblom, 2008; Kaneita et al., 2009; Morphy et al., 2007). This is probably because of the shared role of neurotransmitters within the brain concerning sleep and the experience of depressive and anxiety symptoms (Holmes et al., 2003; Nestler and Carlezon, 2006). For this reason, treating insomnia effectively reduces the onset or worsening of existing anxiety or depressive symptoms. Conversely, treating mental health issues reduces the likelihood of insomnia (Kaneita et al., 2009). Assessment and treatment should therefore be undertaken for all three conditions in patients diagnosed with either anxiety, or depression, or insomnia (Alvaro et al., 2013).

Quality of sleep is a significant factor regarding psychotic symptoms. Sleep disturbance is thought to contribute to creating and maintaining psychotic symptoms, making it a necessary aspect of treatment for psychosis (Freeman et al., 2015). Sleep can be disrupted by antipsychotic medication, lack of daytime activity and the symptoms of psychosis, particularly at night due to fears of nightmares (Afonso et al., 2011; Hofstetter et al., 2005; Wulff and Joyce, 2011; Michels et al., 2014). Poor sleep is extremely common for people experiencing psychosis, enhancing the severity of their symptoms, emotional upset and cognitive issues (Lunsford-Avery et al., 2015).

Having reviewed the importance of exercise, diet and sleep as factors impacting on mental health, it is clear that their presence is vital for wellbeing. Their inadequacy can also cause severe emotional disturbance. Although their importance is known, they are often given token significance within mental health treatment plans. These factors are also severely undervalued within mental health promotion strategies. A change in service philosophy needs to take place so that mental health professionals address these factors as a means of effectively assisting people experiencing mental health difficulties.

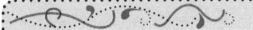

Chapter summary

This chapter began by considering that mental health is often incorrectly viewed as simply an absence of psychiatric symptoms. Rather than being something this simple, it is instead an aspect central to personal health that has to be worked on throughout our lifetime. Service design means professionals dealing with mental and physical health issues normally work independently of each other. This demonstrates a colossal oversight of the reality of patient need, as physical and mental health issues are intrinsically entwined. Until both aspects of health are appropriately valued in each area of care, the effectiveness of physical and mental health treatments will remain limited. The needs of our patients must therefore be placed before those of staff who fail to address care beyond the traditional core business of their individual practice areas.

Further reading and useful websites

MIND (2015) How to improve your wellbeing through physical activity. Available at: **https://www.mind. org.uk/information-support/tips-for-everyday-living/physical-activity-sport-and-exercise/#.WgjM6mi0Pcs**

This MIND document is a useful guide for both practitioners and patients seeking to encourage mental wellbeing through physical health.

Regional Public Health (2012) A guide to promoting health and wellness in the workplace. Available at: **http://www.hauora.co.nz/assets/files/Tools/workplace%20wellness%20resource%20Regional%20 Public%20Health.pdf**

The implementation section of this document provides some useful ideas on improving mental wellbeing within workplaces through exercise, nutrition and a smoke-free environment.

World Health Organization (2004) Promoting mental health. Available at: **http://www.who.int/mental_ health/evidence/en/promoting_mhh.pdf**

Although this is an older document, it is still worth considering because the World Health Organization draws together much useful information on an aspect of health promotion that tends to be under-provided for in practice.

Chapter 2
Common mental health issues

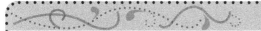
Chapter aims

By the end of the chapter you will be able to:

*   recognise and explain to patients and carers the symptoms of a range of common mental health conditions they may be experiencing;
*   appreciate the significant differences presented within DSM-5 and ICD-10 of the diagnostic criteria regarding serious mental health issues;
*   understand the terminology and stylistic features used within the major diagnostic manuals, questioning or supporting diagnoses applied to the patients we work with;
*   apply a working knowledge of the symptoms of mental illness when assessing the psychological condition of our client group.

Introduction

> ### Case study: Che
>
> *Che knows that he is under surveillance. He has been aware for some time that a CIA team are tracking his movements with satellites because of the implants put into his brain by Russian terrorists. He also knows that mental health services are agents of the state seeking to recover the military secrets the implants contain. The only way that he can keep his thoughts from being read by their thought reading machines is through lining the walls of his flat with foil. Going out is dangerous because of enemy agents, but he is kept safe by the Buddhist angels that walk among us as God's eyes on earth.*

Che's thoughts described in this case study suggest that he is experiencing psychotic symptoms. He is likely to be isolated, scared and untrusting of other people trying to help him. Understanding Che may be difficult because of his unconventional thinking style, and he may be hard to work with because of his distrust of mental health services. He is highly vulnerable and has potential to harm himself or others because of the conviction and content of his deluded beliefs. These factors make Che suitable for assessment for treatment according to the Mental Health Act (1983).

No examination of mental health is complete without a consideration of mental illness. In order to understand mental illness in practice, we need to consider the two major diagnostic categorisation systems currently utilised within international psychiatry. These systems are termed ICD-10 (International Categorization of Diseases Ten) (World Health Organization, 1992) and DSM-5 (Diagnostic and Statistical Manual Five) (American Psychiatric Association, 2013). They provide checklists of symptoms to diagnose a range of mental illnesses. Local policy may dictate the use of either system.

The range of conditions described within DSM-5 and ICD-10 are broad, including both common and rare presentations of mental illness. The diagnoses covered should be treated as viewpoints on mental illness, rather than fact. They are widely accepted in practice as fact, but in reality remain poorly supported by current research. For an overview, see Bentall (2003).

Within this chapter, we consider the conditions commonly encountered in physical and mental healthcare settings. Diagnoses of mental illness covered may be categorised as forms of anxiety, mood disorders, psychosis, eating disorders and personality disorders. DSM-5 and ICD-10 are similar systems but with distinct differences regarding some conditions; therefore each manual will be considered when describing the illnesses they propose. Rather than quoting either manual verbatim, the symptoms described are presented in a format designed for easy understanding by the reader. This chapter therefore represents a user-friendly version of the DSM-5 and ICD-10 texts. In examining the conditions within the diagnostic manuals, DSM-5 will be considered first, with relevant content from ICD-10 presented where it differs. This is because DSM-5 is recently published, and ICD-10 is currently under review for its next edition.

By presenting variations between similar diagnostic criteria, the lack of consensus between ICD and DSM systems is highlighted. This demonstrates how even the basic foundations of psychiatric diagnoses are contentious. Diagnoses are a theoretical viewpoint on mental illness, rather than fact. In practice, generalisations are made that allow patients to fit diagnoses, rather than recognising that individuals are complex and often do not match diagnostic criteria. Although symptoms of mental illness may be observed in practice, diagnoses rely on subjective opinion and patient self-report, which are contentious. The assumption that observable symptoms prove the existence of specific diagnoses is not supported by research evidence. For example, it may be true that patients experience the psychotic symptoms associated with schizophrenia, but this does not mean that a condition termed "schizophrenia" necessarily exists. Therefore, we could argue that symptoms may be reported or observed, but the mental illnesses associated with them do not necessarily exist. In addition, the ability to diagnose conditions proposed by ICD-10 and DSM-5 has limited reliability in practice – this makes it common for patients to be diagnosed with different conditions by individual psychiatrists.

With these aspects in mind, understanding the major diagnostic criteria allows us to question their appropriateness when applied to our patients. This is an important advocacy function of the modern mental health professional because of the potential power imbalance experienced by patients within the psychiatric system. Accurate diagnosis is critical because it determines the course of treatment recommended, therefore its effectiveness for the patient. Knowledge of diagnostic criteria allows an appreciation of its accuracy when applied in practice, therefore supports challenge of inappropriate treatment.

Anxiety disorders

Anxiety disorders are numerous and differ considerably in presentation. They include agoraphobia, obsessive-compulsive disorder, hoarding disorder, generalised anxiety disorder (GAD), social anxiety disorder (SAD) and panic attack specifier (PA). We will examine the latter three of these conditions as examples of common anxiety disorders.

Generalised anxiety disorder

DSM-5 suggests that GAD may be diagnosed if a person experiences anxiety beyond their control within multiple aspects of their life. ICD-10 terms this experience of persistent and generalised anxiety as "free floating" because it does not apply to any set situation or emotion. Anxiety must not be due to taking of substances, or as a result of any other physical or mental condition. Anxiety must occur "more days than not for at least six months" and cause "clinically significant distress". Adults must experience at least three, and children at least one, of these symptoms:

1. Feeling restless or on edge.
2. Tiring easily.
3. Issues with concentration.

4. Being irritable.

5. Muscular tension.

6. Disturbed sleep.

(Adapted from DSM-5, 300.02)

ICD-10 does not specify numbers of symptoms required for a diagnosis of GAD to be made, and describes them differently from the presentation made in DSM-5. They vary but may include:

1. Persistent nervousness.

2. Trembling.

3. Irritability.

4. Sweating.

5. Lightheadedness.

6. **Palpitations**.

7. Dizziness.

8. Abdominal discomfort.

9. Regular fear that the patient or a relative will become ill or have an accident.

(Adapted from ICD-10, F41.1)

These definitions differ but do not directly contradict each other. With GAD, worry appears as bodily sensations, there being more emphasis on symptoms relating to tiredness in DSM-5 than ICD-10. Both systems describe a person whose physical wellbeing is disturbed by their thinking. They will appear distracted, unenthusiastic and irritable. They will be uninterested in social interaction except perhaps to complain about their worries or the actions of other people. Enthusiasm for change and optimism about addressing their anxiety issues are likely to be low. The person may appear physically drained and low in mood.

It is interesting to note that the underlying cause of GAD – maladaptive thought patterns – are not included as symptoms within these definitions. Both GAD and social anxiety disorder (SAD) are presented in this way, despite the thought processes common to anxiety conditions being central to their creation and maintenance (Manning and Ridgeway, 2016).

Social anxiety disorder

SAD is presented by DSM-5 as:

1. A persistent ("typically lasting for six months or more") disproportionate fear of social situations due to concerns of negative judgement by others in these settings. For children, this must occur when interacting with other children.

2. Specific social situations are either actively avoided or endured with "intense fear".

3. Distress caused is "clinically significant" or impairs the person's usual functioning.

4. Fears are not a result of taking substances, or of other physical or mental conditions.

(Adapted from DSM-5, 300.23)

Although it does not list SAD, ICD-10 presents social phobia as an equivalent condition. This is described as a fear of scrutiny by others, leading to an avoidance of social situations. ICD-10 furthers our understanding of the condition by suggesting that patients experiencing it are likely to have self-esteem issues and are unduly concerned about criticism. They often mistake symptoms of anxiety with the cause of the issue (e.g. "I am nervous because I keep blushing"), rather than recognising their **physiological** symptoms as the result of feeling anxious. Additional symptoms of anxiety highlighted by ICD-10 include:

1. Blushing.

2. Hand tremor.

3. **Nausea**.

4. Urgency of urination.

(Adapted from ICD-10, F40.1)

A person experiencing SAD will find attending specific social events extremely threatening. This can result in fears of speaking to new people, or fears of interaction with well known family or friends. An observer experiencing the same social situation may find these fears difficult to understand. DSM-5 describes the condition's features, but does not specify the thought patterns underpinning this disorder. This omission makes little sense if we consider how SAD develops and is maintained in practice.

Case study: Anxiety issues

Kelly has been referred for treatment by her GP to a local community mental health service due to suspected social anxiety disorder. She is a 19-year-old woman who is the parent of Conner, a 2-year-old boy. She describes herself as having always been quiet, but over the last year has become more socially withdrawn. After separating from her partner last year, Kelly moved back to her parents' home, and left her job following a panic attack. She says she does not leave the house unless she has to because she is worried about having further panic attacks. Kelly is unsure what caused her to panic, but thinks it was due to being surrounded by people, and knowing that they might ask her questions she couldn't answer. When asked to describe her experience further, Kelly finds it difficult to do so because "it's a bit of a blur", but is able to recall that she felt lightheaded and sick, her heart was racing, and she was blushing without knowing why. She is tearful in recalling these events, says that she feels worried and very tense, and keeps thinking "how stupid it all is". She also says that she would like to get back to work, meet a new partner and get her own flat again, "because this would be much better for me and Conner".

This example of SAD highlights the overlapping nature of anxiety conditions, which commonly include panic attacks.

Panic attack specifier

PA is not a separate disorder in DSM-5. It is, however, presented as a distinct condition by ICD-10 as Panic Disorder. DSM-5 suggests PA is potentially associated with every listed anxiety disorder. It may also occur in people experiencing mental and physical health conditions other than anxiety. PA is therefore a "specifier" added to other conditions, e.g. major depressive disorder with panic attacks.

PA is described by DSM-5 as an abrupt intense surge of fear peaking after a few minutes. It may occur either from a state of anxiety or calm. It is diagnosable through the simultaneous occurrence of four or more of these symptoms:

1. **Tachycardia**.
2. Sweating.
3. Shaking.
4. **Hyperventilation**.
5. Feeling choked.
6. Chest pain.
7. Nausea.
8. Feeling faint.
9. Feeling chilled or hot regardless of external temperature.
10. Tingling sensations or feeling numb.
11. Feeling detached from reality.
12. Fear of insanity.
13. Fear of imminent death.

(Adapted from DSM-5, 300.01)

Symptoms listed by ICD-10 for panic disorder are:

1. Sudden palpitations.
2. Chest pain.
3. Choking sensations.
4. Dizziness.
5. Feelings of unreality.
6. Fear of death, loss of control, or insanity.

(Adapted from ICD-10, F41.0)

The symptoms listed by DSM-5 and ICD-10 are varied but inter-related. They are deeply threatening in their unpredictability and are consequently frightening to the person experiencing them. Because of this, they act as a powerful incentive to avoid feared situations. As with other aspects of anxiety, neither diagnostic system describes the cognitive elements that cause and maintain PA. This aspect is worth considering further through a re-evaluation of Kelly's situation in Activity 2.1.

Activity 2.1   *Critical thinking*

Having explored some examples of common anxiety conditions, consider the case example of Kelly (p. 21).

Does the information available to you suggest that she is experiencing a social anxiety disorder as her GP suggests? If not, would another form of diagnosis be more appropriate?

What, if any, additional information would you like to gather from her?

What motivating factors would you highlight if you were to work with Kelly on this issue?

A suggested answer is presented at the end of this chapter.

Reviewing Kelly's situation in Activity 2.1 highlights the overlap between related conditions. This factor is relevant when we consider that DSM-5 and ICD-10 present anxiety and mood disorders separately. This is misleading because the co-morbidity of these conditions is considerable – few people experiencing one do not also experience the other (Coplan et al., 2015). With this in mind, we will now consider common examples of mood disorders.

Mood disorders

Mood disorders listed by DSM 5 include persistent depressive disorder (dysthymia) (PDD), major depressive disorder (MDD), bipolar I (BD I) and bipolar II (BD II) disorders. The conditions included as mood disorders are few in number but not in complexity. Our discussion begins with **dysthymia** as the least severe of mood disorders and as a basis for examining major depression and bipolar disorders. DSM-5 accepts the subjective report of the patient or practitioner observation as evidence of symptoms of these conditions.

Persistent depressive disorder (dysthymia)

For a diagnosis of PDD, DSM-5 requires an adult to have experienced depressed mood most of the day for more days than not over the last two years. A child is required to have experienced depressed mood or irritability most of the day for more days than not over at least the last year. The person may not have been symptom-free for periods of more than two months during this time, and their symptoms of PDD must cause impairment in functioning, or clinically significant distress. In addition, at least two of these symptoms must occur:

1. Disturbed appetite.

2. Disturbed sleeping pattern.

3. Lack of energy.

4. Poor self-esteem.

5. Difficulty concentrating or decision-making.

6. Hopelessness.

(Adapted from DSM-5, 300.4)

DSM-5 stipulates that PDD may not be the result of another mental or physical health condition, or due to taking substances. This diagnosis is inappropriate if the patient has previously experienced mania, hypomania or cyclothymic disorder (the presence of mild bipolar symptoms).

A person experiencing PDD may experience periods of remission, when they feel more focused and energised than usual. Remission can occur either during each day, or over longer time periods. However, the person will more often than not remain distracted from present circumstances. They may favour their own company and a sedentary lifestyle rather than busy activity with other people. Sleeping issues make them likely to rise late and remain awake late at night; if they are employed, they may be regularly off work on health grounds. They are likely to be overweight due to poor diet and lack of exercise, but alternatively could be underweight due to lack of appetite. Their relationships with others are likely to be limited due to their lack of enthusiasm for life and interest in their environment. Feelings of hopelessness and low self-esteem make PDD a chronic condition where the person finds change hard to imagine, plan and activate.

PDD is a long-term, relatively mild condition when compared to other mood disorders. It differs considerably from major depressive disorder (MDD), which is characterised by a more severe onset, and is diagnosable after a short period of time.

Major depressive disorder

DSM-5 presents MDD as the presence of five or more symptoms causing functional impairment or clinically significant distress, which must include depressed mood or diminished interest:

1. Most of almost every day spent experiencing depressed mood.

2. Most of almost every day experiencing little interest in most activities.

3. Change in weight of 5% or more in a month, or changes in appetite almost daily.

4. Insomnia or **hypersomnia** almost daily.

5. Observable agitation or **psychomotor retardation** almost daily.

6. Fatigue almost daily.

7. Feeling inappropriately guilty or worthless almost daily.

8. Inability to concentrate or make decisions almost daily.

9. Suicide plans, a suicide attempt, or recurrent thoughts of suicide or death.

(Adapted from DSM-5, 296.32)

ICD-10 confirms these symptoms under the diagnostic category of recurrent depressive disorder, adding loss of **libido** to this list. To receive a diagnosis of MDD within DSM-5, symptoms cannot be attributable to another physical or mental condition, or due to taking substances. This diagnosis is prohibited if the patient has previously experienced mania or hypomania. MDD is distinguished from a major depressive episode caused by grief. Grief is a healthy process characterised by waves of emotion, including some positive ones, resulting from thoughts of the loss; the MDD experience is persistently negative, and features self-loathing generally absent in grief.

Unlike DSM-5, ICD-10 does not state for how long or how frequently low mood must occur within MDD. ICD-10 categorises severity of depressive episodes and the presence or absence of psychosis as separate categories of depression. Mild depressive episodes occur when:

1. Two or three symptoms of depression are present.

2. The person is able to continue with most necessary activities.

Moderate depressive episodes include:

1. At least four symptoms of depression.

2. Great difficulty in completing everyday activities.

For a diagnosis of a severe depressive episode:

1. There cannot have been previous manic episodes.

2. Several symptoms of depression are severe and cause distress.

3. Feelings of worthlessness, low self-esteem and guilt are common.

4. Thoughts and acts of suicide are common.

5. Physical symptoms of depression (e.g. agitation, weight loss, sleeping issues) usually occur.

(Adapted from ICD-10, F32)

Overlap between DSM-5 and ICD-10 categorisations of more severe forms of depression are therefore considerable. ICD-10 allows diagnosis of considerably less severe presentations, which may have significant impact on treatment provided.

The person experiencing MDD is socially withdrawn and highly uncommunicative. When they do speak, they are likely to be fixated on their own highly negative viewpoint. They may actively discuss thoughts of suicide, or keep them hidden. Attempts to cheer them up are likely to be ineffective because these sentiments will seem entirely unrealistic to the patient. People who have recovered from MDD describe their minds as "racing" rather than being underactive, so it is important to remember this when attempting to communicate with them. These features should be noted when considering James's case study.

Case study: Concerns regarding depression

James is a 17-year-old student currently studying for his A-levels. He has few close friends, describing himself as "a loner". He attends school daily, consistently gaining good grades, but rarely if ever contributes in class discussions. When not at school, James spends his time in his bedroom searching the internet. His parents are concerned that he is too thin and that they "no longer know him" because he is so different from the outgoing boy he used to be. James's mother believes that he may be depressed because he refuses to eat with the rest of his family, rarely speaks to them, and "always dresses in miserable colours".

This description of James's situation suggests that further assessment is warranted regarding his current state of mental wellbeing. These aspects are explored further within Activity 2.2.

Activity 2.2   *Team working*

Imagine that you are part of a Child and Adolescent Mental Health (CAMHS) team. Following a request from his mother, James is referred to the team for assessment and treatment. One of your colleagues is dismissive of this referral, saying, "We shouldn't be working with this boy because what he is experiencing is a normal part of growing up." Another of your colleagues refutes this view, saying that he feels James needs to be seen urgently because he poses a significant risk of developing depression. These opposing views cause some debate within the team, particularly because the service has a long waiting list making it impossible to work with every person referred for treatment.

What are your views on the issues being experienced by James, and how much of a priority is it for CAMHS to work with him at this time?

A suggested answer is presented at the end of this chapter.

James's example illustrates that despite the specificity of diagnostic categories presented by DSM-5 and ICD-10, potential for debate exists regarding all clinical presentations. Having examined the MDD diagnosis, we can now consider the meaning of bipolar disorder I and II. Close attention must be paid to the terminology used within these conditions as they are potentially confusing.

Bipolar I disorder

DSM-5 specifies that a diagnosis of bipolar I disorder (BD I) requires the patient to meet the criteria required for a manic episode (ME). This is distinct from a hypomanic episode (HE);

HE and major depressive episodes (MDE) are common in BD I but are not sufficient alone, or required for a diagnosis to be made, as they do not always occur. As well as requiring the presence of an ME, an MDE must also include criteria for MDD (p. 24), except that these depressive symptoms are not the person's norm.

Manic episode

An ME is defined by DSM-5 as a period of at least a week when most of almost every day includes consistently abnormal irritable or elevated mood, featuring "persistently goal-directed activity or energy". Symptoms must impair function, or require hospitalisation due to psychotic features, or for the safety of the person or others. Differences in diagnosis concerning ME apply for people with elevated mood compared to those experiencing irritability. During this period, a patient with elevated mood requires at least three changes from their usual behaviour to justify a diagnosis of ME. For a patient with irritable rather than elated mood, four changes are required from their usual behaviour. Examples of potential changes to behaviour are:

1. **Grandiose** self-importance and unrealistically exaggerated self-esteem.
2. Reduced need for sleep.
3. Becoming much more talkative or feeling unable to stop speaking.
4. Experiencing racing thoughts or limited logic in connections between ideas.
5. Being highly distracted by apparently irrelevant external stimuli.
6. Physical agitation or increased goal-orientated activity.
7. Undertaking high-risk activities that are out of character.

(Adapted from DSM-5, 296.41)

Symptoms may not be attributable to another physical or mental condition, or as the result of taking substances. These symptoms may be replaced at times with an HE or MDE occurring instead. Having examined the ME requirements of bipolar I disorder, it makes sense to next consider a variant of this condition, bipolar II disorder.

Bipolar II disorder

DSM-5 requires the patient diagnosed with BD II to meet the criteria for a past or current major depressive episode, and a current or past hypomanic episode. BD II therefore differs from BD I because both manic and depressive episodes are required in BD II; within BD I they may occur, but only mania is necessary. The severity of impact on individual functioning is less in hypomania compared to a manic episode.

Hypomanic episode

The criteria for a hypomanic episode is identical to that of a manic episode (above) except that:

1. The period of disturbance from usual behaviour is at least four, rather than seven days.

2. It is not necessary to hospitalise the person, and their functioning is not significantly impaired.

3. Psychotic features may not occur with this diagnosis.

(Adapted from DSM-5, 296.41)

ICD-10 presents hypomania identically to hypomanic episodes in DSM-5, except that irritability may feature instead of euphoria. Although HE symptoms may present very similarly to an ME, the person experiencing them is able to continue relatively normally during periods of hypomania. However, care must be exercised with BD II patients due to the impact of depression, a factor that is not necessarily the case with BD I patients.

Experiences of mania may include elation; however, patients in recovery from BD I and II report that the condition is more often a confusing, frightening one of extreme agitation. It is therefore potentially inaccurate to assume mania is a happy or "high" experience. Particular care must be taken in supporting people during periods of depression, as suicide risk may increase following change from a state of mania (Stange et al., 2016).

The presentation of people with bipolar disorder may change radically over a period of time. They may experience extended periods where symptoms remain controlled. At other times they may experience severe depressive or manic episodes. Individual presentations vary, so it is impossible to predict on each occasion if the person will recover to a state of relative calm, or instead fluctuate between mania and depression.

The diagnostic criteria of mania is confusing because it is so broad. A person who is manic may appear childlike and playful, or may be demanding and arrogant, depending on their individual presentation. Some people while manic are gregarious, enjoying meeting new people and having new experiences they would not consider when asymptomatic. This may result in feelings of regret or guilt when the person is no longer manic because of the impact that their spending or sexual activity have on existing relationships with other people. Speaking with a manic person who is experiencing symptoms of mania is difficult because they tend to present their own views rather than taking into account those of other people; they may be repetitive, or make cognitive leaps during conversations that are unclear to others.

Having reviewed mood disorders, it is natural to now examine psychosis because of the overlap of symptoms between categories.

Psychosis

Psychosis is both a feature of other mental illnesses (for example, bipolar I disorder) and a major categorisation of mental disorder. Examples of psychotic conditions include **catatonia**, substance/medication-induced psychotic disorder, schizophrenia, brief psychotic disorder and schizoaffective disorder (SD). Although all are significant conditions, we will examine the last three of these as key psychotic presentations.

Schizophrenia

Schizophrenia is a diagnosis approached by DSM-5 and ICD-10 in very different fashions. DSM-5 describes one broad condition, whereas ICD-10 presents seven categories of schizophrenia. DSM-5 requires the presence "for a significant proportion of time" over a month, of two or more of these criteria:

1. **Delusions**.

2. Hallucinations.

3. Disorganised speech.

4. Catatonic or "grossly disorganised" behaviour.

5. "Negative symptoms" – poor self-care, low mood, social withdrawal.

(Adapted from DSM-5, 295.90)

A DSM-5 diagnosis of schizophrenia must include either delusions, hallucinations or disorganised speech. Interpersonal functioning must have been significantly reduced for "a significant portion of time" compared to before the condition. Over a six-month period there must be the presence of negative symptoms, or the presence at reduced levels of at least two categories of delusions, hallucinations or disorganised speech. Symptoms cannot be attributable to another physical or mental condition, or as the result of taking substances.

Having considered the DSM-5 diagnosis of schizophrenia, the ICD-10 approach to multiple classification of the condition can be considered. Catatonic, paranoid, hebephrenic, residual, simple, undifferentiated schizophrenia and post-schizophrenic depression are individually categorised by the ICD-10 system.

Catatonic schizophrenia is characterised by:

1. **Psychomotor** disturbance – potentially alternating between lack of movement and automatic obedience to commands by others.

2. Unusual postures held for long periods of time.

3. Periods of extreme excitement (this may not feature).

4. Vivid hallucinations and a dreamlike state may be experienced.

(Adapted from ICD-10, F20.2)

Paranoid schizophrenia features:

1. Delusions that remain fixed and are often paranoid.

2. Auditory hallucinations.

3. Perceptual disturbances.

4. An absence or limited disturbances of mood, decision-making ability, speech, or catatonia.

(Adapted from ICD-10, F20.0)

Hebephrenic schizophrenia is normally only diagnosed in adolescents or young adults. It is characterised by these symptoms:

1. Negative, shallow and inappropriate mood.

2. Loss of decision-making ability.

3. Experiences of delusions and hallucinations that are fleeting and fragmentary.

4. Unpredictable and irresponsible behaviour.

5. Stereotyped mannerisms of schizophrenia.

6. Disorganised thoughts.

7. Incoherent speech.

8. Social isolation.

(Adapted from ICD-10, F20.1)

A diagnosis of residual schizophrenia may be given where a person's symptoms change from psychotic to mainly "negative". These are defined as:

1. Slowing of movements and underactivity.

2. Lack of expressed emotion.

3. Lack of initiative and passivity.

4. Limited speech in terms of content and frequency; the person may struggle to interact effectively with others.

5. Nonverbal communication that confuses or limits understanding by others (for example, tone and volume of voice do not match content expressed).

6. An absence of self-care (not washing, wearing dirty clothes, losing or gaining weight).

(Adapted from ICD-10, F20.5)

Simple schizophrenia is described as a gradual development of:

1. Behaviour that is viewed by others as highly unusual, illogical or strange.

2. An inability to meet the demands of society.

3. A decline in interpersonal performance.

4. The loss of emotional response and decision-making abilities without the presence of psychotic symptoms.

(Adapted from ICD-10, F20.6)

Post-schizophrenic depression (ICD-10, F20.4) occurs when limited symptoms of schizophrenia remain, becoming less prominent than symptoms of depression. Increased awareness of their condition may account for increased suicide risk within this patient group. A patient diagnosed with undifferentiated schizophrenia (ICD-10, F20.3) will display symptoms from more than one subtype without clearly meeting a full set of characteristics.

ICD-10 lists the major delusional experiences of schizophrenia as:

1. Thought echo (a delusion that the person's thoughts can be heard out loud).

2. Thought insertion (a delusion that the person's thoughts are not their own, being inserted into their mind by an external force or person).

3. Thought withdrawal (a delusion that the person's thoughts are being removed from their mind by an external force or person).

4. Thought broadcasting (a delusion that the person's thoughts are being delivered into the mind of some or all other people).

5. Delusional perception (a delusion where routine events are given false meanings – for example, the slogan on another person's t-shirt is a message from another universe).

6. Delusions of control (a delusion that the person's thoughts, feelings or behaviours are under control of other people or external forces).

7. Hearing voices (hallucinations of voices talking about the person in the third person).

8. Thought disorder (illogical, bizarre or deluded thoughts observable through disorganised speech).

(Adapted from ICD-10, F20)

Unless they experience incoherence in speech, a person diagnosed with schizophrenia will be able to engage in superficial conversation, but may become distrustful when subjects of particularly personal relevance are discussed. Their delusions are bizarre and fixed, meaning logic has very little impact. Delusions often involve paranoid, religious or supernatural subject matters and may be persecutory in nature. **Hallucinations** may affect any of the senses but are most commonly auditory. They can be supportive, but are normally persecutory towards the person experiencing them. Auditory hallucinations may command the person to act out thoughts they do not wish to undertake – in extreme circumstances, this may be to attack another person or to kill themselves. An inward focus may result in the person appearing detached from the world; they may undertake incomprehensible ritual behaviours, or appear dishevelled or unkempt. With these factors in mind, consider Mary's case study.

Case study: Psychotic symptoms

Mary is a woman in her fifties who has received regular treatment from mental health services since her late teens. She has always lived independently, but regularly requires intervention following periods where she loses weight rapidly.

Mary is usually cooperative in her treatment, including washing, changing her clothes and eating meals provided for her. She is able to discuss practical issues such as where she wants to live, and gives consent to attend therapeutic groups and to taking medication when in hospital. On occasion Mary

(continued)

continued . . . . •

appears to be incomprehensible, speaking rapidly and with little logical progression between sentences. The nature of her speech is predominantly religious; at these times Mary describes herself as several different biblical characters including Mary Magdalene, St Paul and Jesus. She does not report hearing voices, but has stated that in the past God has spoken to her in dreams. Mary is thought to have made a serious suicide attempt during her twenties but has not reported suicidal thoughts to staff working with her in recent years.

Having read about Mary's situation, it is now possible to consider the process of working with her.

Activity 2.3   *Decision-making*

Imagine you are working in an inpatient unit where Mary has been informally admitted for treatment following a period of apparent religious delusions and severe weight loss. Because of her ongoing regularity of admission to inpatient care, you are asked to under-take a review of her condition. From the information you have about her, what sort of diagnosis do you feel is indicated?

A suggested answer is presented at the end of this chapter.

Diagnosing Mary is difficult due to the limited information available to us. The presentation of schizophrenia is varied, but often extreme in nature. Symptoms can cause severe disablement and suffering in those experiencing them, and can result in early death through unhealthy life-style or suicide. Having reviewed schizophrenia, we can appreciate the differences between this condition and brief psychotic disorder.

Brief psychotic disorder

The criteria presented in DSM-5 for brief psychotic disorder is identical to schizophrenia except that it does not include the presence of negative symptoms, and symptoms last between a day and a month. The ICD-10 equivalent to brief psychotic disorder is acute schizophrenia-like psychotic disorder. There is no suggestion made in DSM-5 that the severity of this condition is any less than in schizophrenia; ICD-10 specifies the condition has symptoms of comparable severity to schizo-phrenia. Complete recovery must occur "within a few months, often within a few weeks or days" for a diagnosis to be valid.

Schizoaffective disorder

DSM-5 presents schizoaffective disorder as "an uninterrupted period of illness" (length unspec-ified) where criteria for schizophrenia are met simultaneously with either major depressive disorder (as long as the symptom of depressed mood is met) or mania. There must be a current or historic period of two or more weeks where delusions or hallucinations occur without major depressive disorder or mania. However, MDD or mania must be present "for the majority of the total duration" when the schizophrenic criteria are both being met and in remission. Symptoms cannot be attributable to another physical or mental condition, or as the result of taking substances. ICD-10 presents schizoaffective disorder as separate manic and depressive subtypes.

The boundaries between psychosis and mood disorders are fluid in the case of schizoaffective disorder. The person experiencing this condition undergoes a greater range of distressing symptoms than those diagnosed with schizophrenia, bipolar disorder I or II, or major depressive disorder. This is a complex presentation and may as a consequence be difficult to treat effectively. It is also likely to cause considerable misery to the patient, putting them at increased risk of suicide. This is also true of eating disorders, the next area for consideration.

Eating disorders

The eating disorders listed within DSM-5 include avoidant/restrictive food intake disorder, anorexia nervosa (AN), bulimia nervosa (BN) and binge-eating disorder (BED). The latter three diagnoses are considered further as the major examples of eating disorders.

Anorexia nervosa

DSM-5 defines AN as diagnosable when these characteristics are present:

1. A body weight that is "less than minimally normal" in adults, or "less than minimally expected" in children as a result of dietary intake.
2. Continued extreme fear of weight gain despite being clearly underweight.
3. Inability to recognise issues resulting from being clearly underweight, or to realistically appraise personal bodyweight.
4. The patient's view of themselves is determined almost entirely by body shape or weight.

(Adapted from DSM-5, 307.1)

Although expressed in a different fashion, ICD-10 criteria can be seen to overlap with DSM-5 diagnosis. ICD-10 additionally allows a diagnosis of **atypical** AN if most required symptoms of the condition are met, but some features are not fully present. For example, having a realistic awareness of their appearance when severely underweight.

AN is presented in DSM-5 according to restricting or binge-eating/purging subtypes. AN restricting type occurs when over the last three months the person has maintained or lost weight through exercise or restricted dietary intake only, rather than purging through vomiting, use of enemas, diuretics or laxatives. AN binge-eating/purging type requires the person to repeatedly binge eat and purge over a three-month period. Severity of anorexia nervosa is defined by DSM-5 according to body mass index (BMI) scores as: mild (BMI over 17); moderate (BMI of 16 to 16.99); severe (BMI of 15 to 15.99) and extreme (BMI of less than 15). DSM-5 allows adjustment of severity of categorisation according to "other symptoms and the degree of functional disability".

A person with AN will be fixated on achieving and maintaining a very low body weight, so attempts to reassure them that they are already thin are ineffective. The condition is associated with low self-esteem, with patients attempting to improve their self-worth through maintaining extremely low body weight. Self-report of childhood abuse of various forms is high for people with this diagnosis. Until they engage with the recovery process, a patient experiencing symptoms of anorexia nervosa may be secretive about their dietary intake, exercise and purging. It is incorrect to think of it involving restricted diet only, as there are clear overlaps with the purging behaviour of bulimia nervosa.

Bulimia nervosa

DSM-5 defines BN as the presence of binge-eating episodes with associated behaviours to prevent weight gain occurring at least weekly over three months. For a DSM-5 diagnosis, these factors must occur:

1. BN behaviours cannot occur exclusively in the presence of anorexia nervosa.
2. The patient's self-evaluation is based almost entirely on body shape or weight.
3. Binge-eating episodes involve consuming much more food than "most individuals would eat" in similar circumstances.
4. The person feels out of control of the volume or type of food they eat during binge-eating episodes.
5. Unhealthy behaviours are used to prevent weight gain, including excessive exercise, vomiting, fasting, use of laxatives or diuretics.

(Adapted from DSM-5, 307.51)

ICD-10 criteria supports DSM-5 diagnostic categorisation. ICD-10 allows a diagnosis of atypical BN when most but not all required symptoms are present. For example, purging may occur without concerns about body weight or shape.

Severity of BN is defined by DSM-5 according to "regularity of inappropriate compensatory behaviours" as: mild (averaging 1–3 times per week); moderate (averaging 4–7 times per week); severe (averaging 8–13 times per week) and extreme (averaging 14 or more times per week). Severity may be adjusted according to "other symptoms and the degree of functional disability".

BN has similarities but also critical differences to AN. Despite extensive concerns with body weight, there is no indication that the person will be underweight, therefore a person experiencing BN may have an above average body mass index. Where the person experiencing AN successfully controls their dietary intake, the person experiencing BN is unable to control the amount of food they consume. This lack of control does not necessarily occur between binges, whereas AN is characterised by persistent control of calorie intake. Both conditions are characterised with low self-esteem focused on physical appearance – typically thoughts such as, "When I look better, I will be a more worthwhile person." Consider factors so far covered in terms of Morowa's situation in the following case study.

··

Case study: Eating issues

Morowa is a 34-year-old woman who is admitted to hospital following a potentially fatal overdose of paracetamol. During her recovery she confides to a member of staff that she makes herself sick after overeating and hates herself because of her weight. She is not deemed detainable under the Mental Health Act (1983) because of improvements in her mood and denial of suicidal intent. She does, however, agree to be monitored in the community because of the seriousness of her overdose.

··

Review relevant factors presented in Morowa's situation when undertaking Activity 2.4.

Activity 2.4   *Decision-making*

Imagine you are Morowa's caseworker. From working with her, it becomes apparent that she justifies her binge-eating through a maladaptive thought process. For example, she says to you: "If I am good and do my aerobics, I deserve to eat a packet of biscuits." She also says that her weight is no-one else's business, that white European staff are racist towards her because her build is due to her Ghanaian heritage, and that her overdose was not linked to her weight.

Considering that Morowa is an informal patient without an official diagnosis, how would you respond to these statements?

A suggested answer is presented at the end of this chapter.

Having considered Morowa's situation and BN in general, it is now possible to examine binge-eating disorder, a related but differing condition.

Binge-eating disorder

ICD-10 does not present an equivalent diagnosis to BED. DSM-5 defines it as binge-eating episodes occurring at least weekly over three months. For a diagnosis, these factors must occur:

1. BED behaviours cannot include associated unhealthy behaviours used to prevent weight gain, or occur exclusively in the presence of AN or BN.

2. The person feels out of control of the volume or type of food consumed during binge-eating episodes.

3. Binge-eating creates considerable distress in the patient.

(Adapted from DSM-5, 307.51)

The severity of BED is defined according to frequency of binge-eating episodes as: mild (1–3 times per week); moderate (4–7 times per week); severe (8–13 times per week) and extreme (14 or more times per week). DSM-5 allows severity to be adjusted according to "other symptoms and the degree of functional disability".

Rather than the simple definition of binge-eating provided in BN as consumption of much more food than "most individuals would eat" in similar circumstances, binge-eating is described for BED in more detail. For a diagnosis to be made, binge-eating episodes must meet at least three of these characteristics:

1. More rapid eating than is "normal".

2. Becoming uncomfortably full through binge-eating.

3. Consuming large amounts of food when not hungry.

4. Embarrassment about amounts of food eaten, leading to eating alone.

5. Feelings of severe guilt, disgust or depression following bingeing.

(Adapted from DSM-5, 307.51)

Without compensatory weight loss behaviours, the person experiencing BED is more likely to be overweight than a person with similarly severe BN. People experiencing BED are disturbed by binging, providing an incentive to enable change. DSM-5 suggests their weight does not determine their self-esteem, representing a less rigid thinking style and therefore amenability to taking responsibility for their future eating behaviour. Self-responsibility is a factor highly relevant to treatment of personality disorders, discussion of which occurs next.

Personality disorders

The term "personality disorder" is often mis-represented in practice as a single condition, rather than a number of differing presentations. This is probably because borderline personality disorder, the most prevalent of these conditions, is often referred to as "personality disorder" rather than by its correct title. Other presentations include avoidant, **histrionic**, **narcissistic**, antisocial and obsessive-compulsive personality disorders.

Borderline personality disorder

DSM-5 suggests five or more of these characteristics indicate a borderline personality disorder (BPD):

1. Desperate avoidance of real or imagined abandonment.

2. Intense and unstable personal relationships, fluctuating between adoring and hating significant others.

3. Extensive and consistently disturbed sense of self-identity.

4. Impulsive risky or self-harming activity (i.e. sexual activity, substance use, spending, binge-eating).

5. Recurrent self-injury, suicide attempts or suicide threats.

6. Unstable mood as a result of disproportionate reactions to life events.

7. Ongoing and extensive feelings of "emptiness".

8. Anger issues – expressed inappropriately, excessively or being outside of personal control.

9. Paranoid thinking or symptoms of dissociation (feeling severely detached from personal feelings and behaviour) occurring at times of stress.

(Adapted from DSM-5, 301.83)

The equivalent diagnosis presented in ICD-10 is emotionally unstable personality disorder (EUPD). The person diagnosed must exhibit:

1. Impulsive tendencies without considering consequences.

2. Unpredictable and erratic mood.

3. A liability for outbursts of emotion and behaviour.

4. Quarrelsome behaviour and conflicts with others, particularly if criticised or prevented in achieving their impulsive desires.

(Adapted from ICD-10, F60.3)

Two types of EUPD are presented by ICD-10 as impulsive and borderline types. Impulsive type EUPD features emotional instability and inability to control impulsive behaviour. Borderline type EUPD features:

1. Disturbed self-image, personal aims and internal preferences.

2. Feeling chronically empty.

3. Personal relationships that are unstable and unhealthily intense.

4. A tendency to undertake self-destructive behaviour, including suicide attempts and threats.

(Adapted from ICD-10, F60.3)

Symptoms of EUPD and BPD differ but largely complement each other. They describe an individual who is desperate to control those they interact with because of personal inadequacies and expectations that other people will reject them. They are likely to be aggressive when challenged, often viewing differences in opinion as personal insult. They may fluctuate between being unduly needy and then disinterested in those they have significant relationships with. They are dissatisfied with life, addressing boredom through risky behaviour, only to regret the consequences. Reactions to problems experienced are likely to be extreme, blaming others rather than admitting personal responsibility. Lack of experience in expressing themselves constructively may result in self-injury or suicide attempts during crisis. Ramon provides an example of a person experiencing symptoms of BPD.

Case study: Borderline personality disorder

Ramon is a 27-year-old man with a diagnosis of borderline personality disorder. He is currently home-less and reports being in physical danger because of debts to a drug dealer. He was admitted to a psychiatric unit following threats to kill himself. Since being in hospital he has repeatedly reported feeling suicidal, asking for additional medication as often as possible. Some staff have felt compelled to provide this for him because they feel physically intimidated by him. He has refused to attend thera-peutic groups and is verbally abusive to staff when they ask him to get up in the morning. There is division in the staff group, some of whom believe he has the right to treatment as a person with a rec-ognised mental health issue, and others who say he is a drug addict taking advantage of the system and doesn't deserve treatment on the unit.

Ramon's situation illustrates the complexity of working with people with BPD. This warrants further consideration through Activity 2.5.

Activity 2.5   *Reflection*

Consider what it must be like to be in Ramon's situation. How do staff comments about him make you feel?

As this is a personal reflection, a suggested answer is not provided at the end of this chapter.

Another type of personality disorder with some similarities to BPD is antisocial personality disorder (APD).

Antisocial personality disorder

APD requires the presence since fifteen years of age of three or more of these symptoms:

1. Repeated law breaking behaviour.
2. Deceitfulness for personal benefit.
3. Impulsiveness.
4. Repeated physical violence towards others.
5. Lack of regard for safety of others or self.
6. Repeated irresponsible behaviour.
7. Remorselessness as a result of harming others.

(Adapted from DSM-5, 301.7)

DSM-5 presents APD as a disorder only diagnosable in people from 18 years of age; they must have been diagnosable with conduct disorder before 15 years of age; and their symptoms are not a result of schizophrenia or bipolar disorder.

ICD-10 describes dissocial personality disorder, a condition similar to APD. For a diagnosis, these characteristics are required:

1. A disregard for meeting common social obligations.

2. A significant lack of concern for others' feelings.

3. Problematic behaviour differing significantly from prevailing social norms.

4. Adverse experiences (including punishment) do not alter the person's problematic behaviour.

5. Regular displays of low frustration tolerance.

6. Ease of violence and aggression.

7. Commonly rationalising or blaming others for their problematic behaviour.

(Adapted from ICD-10, F60.2)

A person diagnosed with APD may have previous involvement with criminal justice and mental health services. They may appear confident when meeting new people but seek unequal relationships with others due to a tendency to exploit people. Their impulsivity includes compulsive criminality as a means of meeting short-term personal needs. They may become violent if confronted about their exploitative behaviour, or as a means of guaranteeing their own interests are met.

There are similarities between BPD and APD, in particular lack of genuine relationships, irresponsibility and aggression towards others. These factors are not present in all personality disorders, as we see through considering obsessive-compulsive personality disorder (OCPD) in more detail.

Obsessive-compulsive personality disorder

DSM-5 describes OCPD as a condition occurring by early adulthood that features at least four of these characteristics across a range of contexts:

1. Preoccupation with orderliness within an activity, rather than undertaking it for its original purpose.

2. Inability to complete tasks because of impossible perfectionist tendencies.

3. Personal relationships and leisure activities are de-prioritised as a result of workplace or productivity focus.

4. Lack of flexibility and an over-conscientious outlook regarding moral and ethical issues.

5. Refusal to dispose of worthless objects that have no sentimental value.

6. Inability to delegate tasks/responsibilities to others.

7. Hoarding of money for future disasters.

8. Stubbornness and rigidity in views and behaviours.

(Adapted from DSM-5, 301.4)

A similar condition, described by ICD-10 as anankastic personality disorder, requires these symptoms:

1. Feelings of doubt.

2. Perfectionism.

3. Excessive conscientiousness.

4. Checking and preoccupation with details.

5. Stubbornness.

6. Caution.

7. Rigidity.

8. Insistent thoughts or impulses of less severity than in obsessive-compulsive disorder.

(Adapted from ICD-10, F60.5)

The person experiencing OCPD symptoms finds change difficult because their life is dominated by the habitual nature of the condition. Changing routines will create feelings of dread that are difficult to reason with rationally. This is because ritualised behaviours occur as a result of not dealing with other more threatening issues in the person's life. For example, an unwillingness to face childhood trauma, self-esteem issues or fear of death. When confronted about ritualised behaviours, a person experiencing OCPD symptoms is likely to feel threatened and may become avoidant, tearful or hostile. They tend to find emotional subjects difficult as these aspects of their lives are kept hidden by their ritualised behaviour.

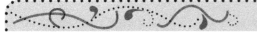

Chapter summary

This chapter has examined examples of the diagnostic criteria provided by DSM-5 and ICD-10 for a range of anxiety and mood disorders, psychosis, eating disorders and personality disorders. These diagnostic manuals provide a useful means of identifying and categorising symptoms of mental ill health. They offer a means of grouping symptoms and setting standards for the diagnosis of mental illness. This makes them invaluable within modern psychiatry as a means of providing a common language between professionals treating serious mental health issues. However, the two main systems examined are not entirely allied in their approach to diagnosing specific issues, creating differences in clinical opinion based around the favoured diagnostic manual being used. Some of the diagnoses are confused and at times contradictory, making their use in practice problematic. A further, more fundamental issue exists regarding the use of diagnostic manuals, namely does the presence of the symptoms observed make the mental health condition represented a reality? This issue fundamentally divides the modern psychiatric system from its critics.

Activities: brief outline answers

Activity 2.1 Critical thinking (page 23)

A SAD diagnosis potentially describes Kelly's condition, but the situation remains unclear as she also exhibits symptoms common to other anxiety disorders. The limitations of a diagnostic system are highlighted here because her situation is more complex than a diagnosis can portray, and more importantly, the cause and potential cure of her symptoms are not provided by either diagnostic system. Another diagnostic category than SAD is therefore unlikely to be of help in describing Kelly's situation.

It is vital that additional information gathering is undertaken with Kelly in a person-centred way, allowing her to describe relevant factors without direction from the assessor. Conversely, undertaking a psychiatric checklist of potential anxiety symptoms may create a biased assessment, missing other non-diagnostic factors in her situation.

Moving from a focus on current problems towards finding solutions is necessary with any form of mental health issue. Kelly provides examples of her ability to work, live independently and experience meaningful relationships. She identifies incentives for change as her son and her desire for independence. These are critical factors when designing positive risk-taking activities with Kelly, so that she can experience anxiety safely and process her panic reactions more realistically in social situations.

Activity 2.2 Team working (page 26)

The issues described need to be considered in context – they could arguably represent teenage development and individualisation; equally, they are indicators of potential depression, and could therefore warrant immediate action. A prompt and considered assessment of James's situation is required based on the views of James and his family. This will allow CAMHS to develop a treatment plan before potential deterioration of the situation.

Activity 2.3 Decision-making (page 32)

More information is required about Mary for a valid diagnosis of her condition. She may be diagnosable with schizophrenia under DSM-5 categorisation, but ICD-10 is more complex, as she could meet the criteria for several schizophrenia subtypes in this system. Bipolar disorder is worthy of consideration as an alternative explanation to schizophrenia. This illustrates the importance of viewing diagnostic categories as guide rather than fact, with no certain answers possible regarding diagnoses.

Activity 2.4 Decision-making (page 35)

Morowa's informal status is important because this means she has the right to refuse any form of treatment. It is vital, however, to challenge her maladaptive thinking as honestly as possible. Her lack of recognition of the connection she previously made between her weight and her suicide attempt is worrying; it would be unfortunate if she had to reach crisis point again before engaging in meaningful discussion of her emotional and mental health. It is important to support Morowa in her treatment choices as a means of building a working relationship with her. Emphasising that we are available when she is ready to talk, rather than trying to force her to talk about her issues, seems a much more effective approach to working with her.

Further reading

The following resources are official guides to understanding the DSM-5 and ICD-10 diagnostic manuals.

American Psychiatric Association (2015) *Understanding Mental Disorders: Your Guide to DSM-5*. Arlington, VA: American Psychiatric Publishing.

Bowie MJ and Schaffer RM (2013) *Understanding ICD-10-CM and ICD-10-PCS: A Worktext*, 2nd edn. Boston, MA: Cengage Learning.

There is also an unofficial guide to understanding DSM-5:

Morrison J (2014) *DSM-5 Made Easy: The Clinician's Guide to Diagnosis*. New York: Guilford Publications.

Useful websites

This is a useful guide to DSM-5 disorders presented by its authors, the American Psychiatric Association:

http://www.dsm5.org/Pages/Default.aspx

This website presents background on the development of the DSM manuals, and highlights changes occurring for the DSM-5 edition:

http://psychcentral.com/dsm-5/

This is ICD-10 in an electronic format, usefully allowing diagnostic review using a portable device:

http://apps.who.int/classifications/icd10/browse/2015/en#/V

Chapter 3
Suicide risk and mental health

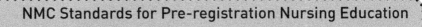

NMC Standards for Pre-registration Nursing Education

This chapter will address the following competencies:

Domain 1: Professional values

2.1 Mental health nurses must practise in a way that addresses the potential power imbalances between professionals and people experiencing mental health problems, including situations when compulsory measures are used, by helping people exercise their rights, upholding safeguards and ensuring minimal restrictions on their lives. They must have an in-depth understanding of mental health legislation and how it relates to care and treatment of people with mental health problems.

Domain 3: Nursing practice and decision-making

7.2 Mental health nurses must work positively and proactively with people who are at risk of suicide or self-harm, and use evidence-based models of suicide prevention, intervention and harm reduction to minimise risk.

Domain 4: Leadership, management and team working

6.1 Mental health nurses must contribute to the management of mental health care environments by giving priority to actions that enhance people's safety, psychological security and therapeutic outcomes, and by ensuring effective communication, positive risk management and continuity of care across service boundaries.

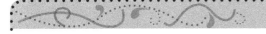

NMC Essential Skills Clusters

This chapter will address the following ESC:

Cluster: Care, compassion and communication

2.10 Recognises situations and acts appropriately when a person's choice may compromise their safety or the safety of others.

2.11 Uses strategies to manage situations where a person's wishes conflict with nursing interventions necessary for the person's safety.

4.4 Upholds people's legal rights and speaks out when these are at risk of being compromised.

8.7 Demonstrates respect for the autonomy and rights of people to withhold consent in relation to treatment within legal frameworks and in relation to people's safety.

> ### Chapter aims
>
> By the end of the chapter you will be able to:
>
> - differentiate between suicide and self-harm, as well as appreciating the links between the two;
> - recognise potential risk factors for suicide while acknowledging the limitations of suicide assessment processes;
> - understand the need to work with patients in an individualised manner to develop their personal suicide prevention strategies;
> - explain the purpose of the most commonly used sections within the Mental Health Act (1983) to staff, patients and relatives.

Introduction

> ### Case study: A death by suicide
>
> *Despite emergency surgery, Akinjide died of his injuries after falling from a cliff near to his home. Passers-by saw him close to the edge and pleaded with him not to jump. Instead, Akinjide smiled and stepped backwards to his death. Witnesses suggested that he looked calm. The post-mortem confirmed that he was not intoxicated at the time of his death.*
>
> *Akinjide had been treated in psychiatric hospitals in different parts of the world from his early twenties until his death at 40. When he died, Akinjide was an informal patient in transition from hospital to community care. He was thought to be in a good state of mind and therefore safe to spend time at home. Staff who worked with him were shocked by his death because he had not given any indication that he wished to kill himself.*

Akinjide's story demonstrates the balance faced by mental health services between concerns for suicide risk, and encouraging service users to take suitable responsibility for their own safety. Although there are many unknown variables in this situation, a more effective suicide risk assessment process may have prevented Akinjide's death.

This chapter considers a wide range of factors linking suicide risk and mental health. It begins by considering suicide methods and the relative risk this decision causes. Next, specific consideration is made to understand reasons why people self-harm. The use of special observations during inpatient admissions are examined as a potential means of reducing suicide risk. Risk factors indicating that a suicide attempt may occur are presented. Our examination includes a consideration of emotional, cognitive, behavioural, historical and social factors, and symptoms. Protective social factors and personal attributes that may prevent suicide attempts are provided. The limitations of suicide risk assessment processes and tools are then considered. Following this, consideration is made of anxiety symptoms as indicators of suicide risk. The chapter concludes by considering the use of the Mental Health Act (1983) (MHA) to manage mental health risk.

Dealing with suicide is a very difficult aspect of being a mental health professional. Activity 3.1 asks us to appreciate the impact on professionals when coping with this event.

Activity 3.1   *Critical thinking*

Consider the events of Akinjide's suicide described above. If you had been a member of staff working with him, how would you feel and what questions would you ask yourself about his death?

A suggested answer appears at the end of this chapter.

The questions posed by Activity 3.1 are difficult to answer. Attempting to answer them indicates the enormity of suicide as a troubling event. The possibility of patients attempting suicide is a fundamental aspect of mental health work. Suicide risk is the main reason for compulsory admission to psychiatric inpatient facilities. Despite this, suicide risk is poorly understood by many practitioners. Accurate assessment of risk is difficult because it requires the individual to objectively assess their own risk. Depending on the nature of their condition, mental health patients may lack the ability to accurately undertake this process. Difficulties in assessment are compounded by a need for the person to willingly share suicidal intentions. Commonly, people who are actively suicidal hide their intentions from health professionals, as they seek to prevent them being carried out. Mental health services have a tendency to prioritise treatment for patients who say they are suicidal, rather than appreciating suicide risk of those who keep their feelings hidden. In this way, opportunities to work with some suicidal patients are missed.

Following recommendations by the peer support group Survivors of Bereavement by Suicide (SOBS), the term "committed suicide" is not used in this chapter. It is seen as offensive by this group because of the connotations of suicide as the "committing" of a crime. This respectful attitude guides our discussion of suicide methods.

Suicide methods

Choice of suicide method is critical in terms of survival rates. The first attempt made by a person may be deadly. Methods termed "lethal means", such as shooting, impact by large motor vehicles or trains, and jumping from heights provide instantaneous means of death. Other methods are more likely to be reversible as they may provide opportunities to save the person, depending on the severity of injury. There are many examples of people who have survived after taking overdoses of medication, cutting their wrists, electrocution, and attempts to drown or deprive themselves of oxygen. Some of these suicidal people have used their survival to reassess and change their lives; others undertake further attempts, some of which are successful.

Cutting and overdose are the most common unsuccessful forms of suicide. If cutting is limited enough to pose no threat of death, it is an example of self-harm rather than a suicide attempt. However, rates of successful suicide by people who undertake repeated non-fatal self-injury are extremely high, being up to 10% within this group. Self-injury should therefore be viewed as a representation of emotional turmoil and suicidal potential within the person. Unfortunately, an assumption of "attention seeking" is commonly made by care staff in these situations, creating a significant communication barrier with many high-risk service users.

Feelings of ambivalence occur when a person doesn't want to live any more but also fears dying. This makes empathising with a person who says they want to kill themselves difficult for some practitioners. Ambivalent self-harming behaviour can be wrongly assumed to indicate that the person is disingenuous in their intent to kill themselves. The nature of factors motivating a person towards suicide are often undisclosed, making the job of predicting suicide particularly difficult. This is important for psychiatric practice, as predictability of suicide is central to motivating psychiatric hospital admissions.

Understanding self-harm

Self-harm is a general term for a range of self-injurious activities. These behaviours vary in severity and regularity, with some participants developing regular ritualised patterns of self-harm. Self-injury includes cutting, burning, swallowing of foreign objects such as razors or batteries, and drinking of poisons such as bleach or oven cleaner. Less commonly self-harm involves insertion of objects into the body, for example razor blades into the anus or vagina. Other unusual forms of self-harm develop according to the individual nature of the patient. Non-lethal self-harm can be a means of preventing more dangerous suicide attempts. It acts as a coping strategy for a person who might otherwise attempt to kill themselves. It is critical when a person ceases self-harming for them to develop alternative, more adaptive methods of reacting to feelings of anxiety.

Self-harm initially seems incomprehensible for many people. Its outlandish nature becomes understandable when considered in the context of more socially acceptable forms of self-injury. For example, alcohol, tobacco and recreational drugs directly damage multiple systems of the body. Drugs prescribed for mental health issues also include significant toxic effects. Choosing to use them when not absolutely necessary is therefore self-injurious. Self-harm can occur by omission, many people creating physical health problems through poor diet and avoidance of regular exercise.

Episodes of self-harm provide a focus for discussion about psychological disturbances in the person's life. Health practitioners should never prohibit self-harm as a coping mechanism because a punitive response may encourage patients to become secretive in their self-injurious behaviour. Self-injury should not be the principle focus of therapeutic conversations or care planning. Instead, root causes of suicidal intent must be explored for psychological healing to take place. When personal exploration of this kind occurs, self-harming as a means of coping with troubling feelings may increase before becoming unnecessary, over time. This type of approach requires considerable skill from the healthcare practitioner, as well as commitment to explore difficult issues from the patient. It is important that members of the healthcare team are prepared to explore suicide motivation as a vital topic of conversation. The belief that discussion of suicidal intent should be avoided because "it puts ideas in the patient's head" is misguided. Without discussing the person's intentions, we have no way of knowing how to help them, leaving them unaided in dealing with their troubling thoughts and dangerous impulses. People who self-harm report that self-injury provides them with an enormous sense of relief from tension, suggesting self-harm is a means of dealing with individual anxiety through altering mood. Insight into why this is the case for an individual can be provided through understanding the thought processes of the person concerned.

Self-harm is a means of self-punishment that may be motivated by guilt concerning traumatic incidents in the person's past. People who self-harm report issues commonly concerning sexual trauma. The location of cuts is unlikely to be random, providing information about the role self-harming takes for the individual. Cuts made to exposed parts of the body are more likely to be noticed, suggesting a desire to make concerns public. Cuts in hidden areas highlight the person's shame about self-harming, and personal need to find more socially acceptable means of coping. A person who ingests or injects cleaning products may feel that past sexual trauma makes them "dirty" with a need to be clean. People who conceal razorblades within bodily cavities report previous sexual violations and fear of further abuse. Swallowing foreign objects may be an unconscious attempt to recreate childhood experience of being looked after by healthcare professionals. Not every form of self-harm provides clues about the person's past, but all indicate a lack of self-worth. Self-harm therefore provides an opportunity to engage with the person therapeutically to create lifestyle changes. Through discussing links between past trauma and present behaviour, the person may be able to reassess the logic of punishing themselves for past events.

Helping a person to understand the motivations to self-harm represents positive change that is possible when they are in a relatively settled state of mind. Prior to this, if a person appears to be at particular risk of killing themselves, special observation may be necessary.

Using special observations during inpatient admissions

Special observations are a regular, planned pattern of observation undertaken in an attempt to help prevent self-harm or suicide attempts. Ironically, special observations can actually create a significant risk. Because patients know when they will next be observed, they also know how long they have alone between observations to hurt themselves. This period has been used successfully to achieve suicide on many mental health units. Special observations highlight that professionals feel these patients are incapable of keeping themselves safe. Ironically, this can have a detrimental effect on their self-esteem and recovery.

A positive aspect of special observations is that it provides a chance to engage meaningfully with the patient in a therapeutic fashion. This is important because special observations are often used for patients who professionals have made little therapeutic progress with. Engagement with this group is critical from an early stage in order to understand individual factors contributing to suicide risk for this individual.

Risk factors indicating that a suicide attempt may be more likely

A wide range of factors increasing suicide risk exist. Examples of these aspects may be present for a person, but this does not mean they will attempt suicide. Equally, they may not be relevant factors for a person who successfully kills themselves. Relative frequency, duration and severity are therefore critical in understanding the importance of suicide risk factors (Miller et al., 1986).

Suicide risk may be increased through emotional, cognitive and behavioural aspects, the person's symptoms, social circumstances and relevant history. Emotional and cognitive factors include feelings of powerlessness, and a lack of belief in their ability to resolve problems (Beck et al., 1997; Cull and Gill, 1998; Perlman et al., 2011). Those who perceive a lack of options other than suicide in challenging situations are at greater risk. This is also true of people experiencing suicidal thoughts or making suicide threats (Beck et al., 1997; Beck et al., 1974; Cull and Gill, 1998; Heisel and Flett, 2006; Hirdes et al., 2000; Kutcher and Chehil, 2007; Linehan, 1981; Miller et al., 1986; Posner et al., 2008). Feelings of loss of personal worth or social standing (Heisel and Flett, 2006; Patterson et al., 1983), the inability or unwillingness to engage with support services (Black, 2013) and the lack of a deterrent to undertake suicide (Centre for Addiction and Mental Health (CAMH), 2011) all increase risk.

Behavioural factors indicating increased suicide risk include suicide-related behaviour (e.g. giving possessions away, seeking out people to say goodbye to) (Beck et al., 1997; Hirdes et al., 2000; Posner et al., 2008). Non-fatal self-harm is another indicator, particularly if it is secretive, a new behaviour for the person or has escalated in seriousness or frequency (CAMH, 2011; Linehan, 1981). Increased substance use (Patterson et al., 1983; Perlman et al., 2011) or withdrawal from addictive drugs (CAMH, 2011) are warning behaviours. In these situations, suicide may be a deliberate option, or occur accidentally through overdose due to reduced tolerance of drugs used. Realistic, organised suicide planning, preparation and access to lethal means may all indicate increased risk (e.g. **stockpiling tablets**, researching or rehearsing methods of suicide, access to chosen suicide methods, specifying timing and sequence of planned suicide) (Beck et al., 1997; Beck et al., 1974; Black, 2013; CAMH, 2011; Hirdes et al., 2000; Kutcher and Chehil, 2007; Miller et al., 1986; Patterson et al., 1983; Perlman et al., 2011). Greater likelihood of death and lower possibility of reprieve increase suicide risk (CAMH, 2011). Finally, withdrawing from previously supportive relationships and wider society should be considered as positive indicators of risk (Perlman et al., 2011).

In terms of historical factors, previous unsuccessful suicide attempts, particularly if the person regrets surviving, indicate increased suicide risk (CAMH, 2011; Heisel and Flett, 2006; Linehan 1981; Perlman et al., 2011). This is also true where a family history of suicide or suicidal behaviour exists – people bereaved by suicide are often at high suicide risk themselves, even many years after their bereavement occurred (Nelson et al., 2010). If the person has made precautions against discovery during previous attempts the risk of future successful suicide is increased. Conversely, attempts to gain help during previous attempts lessen future suicide risk (Beck et al., 1974). People with a history of physical, sexual or psychological trauma (possibly presenting as post-traumatic stress symptoms) are at higher suicide risk (Perlman et al., 2011). Anniversaries of traumatic events present greater immediate risk. Examples include physical or sexual assault, or the death of a partner, child or parent (CAMH, 2011).

Symptoms increasing suicide risk include the presence of severe mental illness – particularly auditory hallucinations commanding the person to kill themselves (Hirdes et al., 2000; Kutcher and Chehil, 2007; Patterson et al., 1983; Perlman et al., 2011). People experiencing symptoms of narcissistic or perfectionist personality disorder traits may be at particular risk when experiencing challenging life events (Black, 2013; Hawgood and De Leo, 2014). This is also true for people experiencing obsessive feelings of hostility or impulsive, risk-taking behaviour (Cull and Gill, 1988; Perlman et al., 2011). Chronic physical illness, particularly with resulting unresolved pain, increases suicide risk (Black, 2013; Kutcher and Chehil, 2007; Patterson et al., 1983; Perlman et al., 2011). Significant changes in a person's usual appearance or mood are warning signs that they may be at increased imminent risk. The presence of excessive anxiety, or when the loss of former interests or motivation for living occurs acts as a similar signal (Perlman et al., 2011). Important questions to ask when assessing suicide risk are: is the person currently capable of acting on their suicidal desires? Is the person motivated enough to act, or prevented from acting due to symptoms of apathy? (CAMH, 2011). Finally, we need to consider the additional risk posed if mental health treatment has been unsuccessful to date (Black, 2013).

Social factors indicating suicide risk include family concerns about the person's safety. Families may provide vital context-specific information that services otherwise remain unaware of (Hirdes et al., 2000). People with limited social support networks are at increased risk (Cull and Gill, 1988; Patterson et al., 1983). Age and gender also affect risk – males, and people aged between 40 and 60 years are more likely to kill themselves (CAMH, 2011; Kutcher and Chehil, 2007). Unemployment, financial difficulties and breakdown of important relationships increase risk (Perlman et al., 2011). If the person is in transition between services – for example, leaving prison, discharge from hospital, or moving from children's to adult services – they are at increased suicide risk (CAMH, 2011; Mulder, 2011). This is also true of people who are currently being treated in a psychiatric hospital (Bleich et al., 2011), or who frequently change their address or are homeless (Black, 2013).

Having reviewed an extensive set of factors that increase suicide risk, let us consider Rubin's situation.

> ### Case study: Rubin
>
> *Rubin is a 57-year-old man who was admitted to an accident and emergency department after being found unconscious by his wife, Nina. He had taken an overdose of nitrazepam and may have died without medical intervention. Rubin is unknown to mental health services. He was unwilling to discuss what happened with hospital staff, asking instead to be left alone. Nina says that Rubin has been much more withdrawn recently and is concerned that he may have gambling debts. She was, however, extremely surprised by his actions and is worried that he will succeed should he try to kill himself again.*

The circumstances experienced by Rubin and Nina are deeply troubling for them. Activity 3.2 asks questions related to Rubin's safety.

> ### Activity 3.2   *Critical thinking*
>
> Consider the circumstances of Rubin's situation. What would you suggest his risk of harming himself to be at this time?
>
> *A suggested answer appears at the end of this chapter.*

Rubin was unknown to mental health services at the time of his overdose. His lack of access to services places him at potentially high suicide risk.

The relationship between greater suicide risk and severe mental health conditions

A massively increased risk of suicide exists for people who have undertaken previous attempts, and for those diagnosed with severe mental health issues. For example, Table 3.1 illustrates that people experiencing major depression or eating disorders are over twenty times more likely to kill themselves than the general population (APA, 2013).

Risk factor	Relative risk multiplier
Previous suicide attempt	38.4
Eating disorders	23.1
Major depression	20.4
Mixed drug abuse	19.2

Bipolar disorder	15.0
Dysthymia	12.1
Obsessive-compulsive disorder	11.5
Panic disorder	10.0
Schizophrenia	8.45
Personality disorders	7.08
Alcohol abuse	5.86

Table 3.1: Relative risk multipliers of suicide in specific disorders

Adapted from work by the Centre for Addiction and Mental Health, 2011.

Table 3.1 shows how many times more likely suicide is for the groups listed compared to the general population. Relative risk for people with mental health diagnoses and previous suicide attempts is remarkably high.

Protective factors thought to reduce suicide rates

Having considered aspects contributing significantly to suicide risk, factors that keep people alive can also be considered. Helping suicidal people to develop the preventative skills and attitudes listed in Table 3.2 should be a major focus of suicide prevention work.

Personal attributes

- Possession of reality testing, problem solving and interpersonal skills (Black, 2013; CAMH, 2015; Miller, 2011). These attributes may initially be limited for people experiencing severe mental health issues.
- Realistic self-worth and a sense of personal identity (Miller, 2011).
- An ability to identify realistic and attainable goals that provide a hopeful future (Black, 2013; Miller, 2011).
- Willingness to pursue purposeful and constructive hobbies and activities (Miller, 2011).
- Possessions of underlying reasons for living outweighing reasons for dying (Miller, 2011).
- Religious or spiritual beliefs that prohibit suicide (CAMH, 2015; Miller, 2011).
- Feelings of responsibility towards other people (CAMH, 2015).
- Fear of the suicidal act (CAMH, 2015).

(Continued)

Table 3.2 (Continued)

> **Social factors**
>
> - Strong social support networks with family and wider community (Black, 2013; CAMH, 2015; Miller, 2011).
> - Availability of timely and effective professional interventions that meet their personal needs and ethical values (Black, 2013; CAMH, 2015; Miller, 2011).
> - Limited access to lethal means at times of crisis (CAMH, 2015).
> - The person lives with their children or is pregnant (CAMH, 2015).
> - Living arrangements that are supportive during times of crisis (CAMH, 2015).

Table 3.2: Suicide prevention factors

Working with service users to help them develop these attributes is critical for their long-term development, and ability to reduce input required from mental health services. The significance of these actions is highlighted through consideration of the limitations apparent within suicide risk assessment processes.

The limitations of suicide risk assessment processes

Despite an awareness of known risk factors, the ability to objectively identify signs of suicidal intent is limited. Although symptoms of severe mental ill health suggest a significantly increased risk of those experiencing them undertaking suicide, the presence of such symptoms does not mean an attempt will actually take place. For suicide risk assessment to be effective, more is required than simply identifying the presence of risk. The patient must be understood in a wider context, with emphasis placed on appreciating their individual circumstances, and working with them to develop alternatives to suicide. Following the use of a suicide assessment tool, an informal, ongoing process of suicide risk assessment should be undertaken through regular therapeutic interaction. This process should build rapport, trust and shared understanding of the person's situation. Honest conversation that includes suicide risk, but also explores wider aspects of life, provides both personalised assessment and a process of healing for the **traumatised** individual.

A number of misapprehensions exist concerning the ability of health professionals to predict suicide risk. These include an assumption that the presence of identified risk factors indicates that suicide is likely; that we can categorise individuals as belonging to high or low suicide risk groups; and that suicide rates will reduce if we increase the amount of resources provided to work with high risk groups. Completed suicides are often assumed to have been preventable if risk assessments had been completed more effectively. None of these misapprehensions are supported by research (Mulder, 2011).

An explanation of risk aversion that predominates within mental health services is the need by practitioners to avoid anxiety-provoking decisions concerning suicide risk. Low tolerance to potential suicide risk develops "just in case something happens". Despite understanding the benefits of positive risk-taking, staff tend to focus instead on their own fears of litigation and being blamed if suicide occurs. Without positive risk, patients are encouraged to avoid making decisions that involve facing their fears.

Best practice requires a full range of mental health interventions rather than treatment focused only on the prevention of self-harm. Suicide risk assessment therefore represents a major aspect of treatment, but must not be allowed to become the predominant driver shaping patient care. By working with patients to understand their problems and identify their goals for change, we can reduce suicide risk through meeting individual holistic need. This approach contrasts with unrealistic attempts to predict and prevent suicide, instead encouraging rational clinical decisions based on individual need (Bleich et al., 2011). These contrasting approaches may be kept in mind when considering Jo-Jo's situation.

Case study: Assessing risk

Jo-Jo is a woman in her late twenties with a diagnosis of borderline personality disorder. She has been in regular contact with mental health services since being a teenager and has undertaken a number of suicide attempts. She regularly cuts her arms with razor blades. In the past she has experienced mental health inpatient treatment following threats of suicide. On this occasion, Jo-Jo is detained by police officers using section 136 of the Mental Health Act. Following an assessment under section 12 of the Act, the mental health team discharge Jo-Jo with ongoing support from her existing mental health community practitioner. Jo-Jo responds by saying that she will kill herself if discharged. The team's decision remains unchanged.

Jo-Jo's situation demonstrates a difficult decision when working with a person who self-harms. Here, police officers act to protect a vulnerable member of the public from harming herself, but the mental health assessment team discharge Jo-Jo from their care. Activity 3.3 asks you to consider these actions further:

Activity 3.3   *Critical thinking*

Consider the actions of the mental health assessment team described above. What are the benefits of the decision to discharge Jo-Jo?

A suggested answer is provided at the end of this chapter.

A key skill in making this type of discharge decision is the ability of care staff to determine suicide risk. This is a complex skill; one approach to doing so is through using a suitable suicide risk assessment tool.

The use of suicide risk assessment tools

Numerous suicide risk assessment instruments are available, some being free of charge. Examples of commonly used frameworks are listed on pages 63–4 at the end of this chapter. A number of these instruments are available via request to the authors; where available, contact details are provided.

A major misunderstanding in assessing suicide risk occurs through an over-emphasis on the usefulness of scores produced. Risk assessment scores are one piece of evidence in each individualised mental health situation. Nominal scores for something as subjective as suicide risk have limited value; despite this, it remains common practice for mental health professionals. Within a strongly **risk-averse** mental health practice culture, clinical decisions based on risk assessment scores are preferred because they represent expert opinion.

Arguably, risk assessment scores guide practitioners in determining severity of risk, and therefore actions necessary to keep patients safe. However, these processes have major drawbacks. Allocating care according to suicide risk scores may result in unnecessary interventions if a false positive (an inaccurately exaggerated assessment of suicide risk) occurs. Conversely, a false negative will result in a suicidal person not receiving necessary services. A shift in focus is required by mental health services to reduce their reliance on suicide risk assessment tools. Instead, they should value ongoing therapeutic conversations that feature, but are not entirely dominated by, risk.

Communication between staff and patient is of greatest importance in understanding need through ongoing, unstructured assessment. Patients respond most significantly to personal relationships with staff, something hindered through using highly structured suicide assessment tools.

Focusing on anxiety symptoms to assess suicide risk

The Hermes Deakin Suicide Risk Assessment tool (HDSRA) (Hermes et al., 2009) takes a different approach to other suicide risk assessment processes. This is because HDRSA indicates the presence of suicide risk factors, rather than presenting a nominal risk level. Unlike other suicide risk assessment scales, the focus of the HDSRA is not on suicidal thoughts reported by the patient, but on the presence of severe anxiety and agitation in combination with other potential suicide risk factors. This is because agitation and anxiety are factors normally present immediately before the completion of many suicides. Table 3.3 lists symptoms of anxiety and agitation to consider when assessing suicide risk.

Anxiety and agitation are recognisable symptoms that can be easily monitored. The importance of these symptoms can be highlighted to family members, carers and healthcare staff working in order to indicate when a person is more likely to undertake a spontaneous suicide attempt. Intervention to ensure personal safety therefore becomes appropriate when patients become severely agitated because of the increased suicide risk this state of being represents

- Anxious mood – excessive worry of feared future events.

- Depressed mood – the person lacks interest and pleasure in things they were previously concerned about.

- Tension – patients may appear to be restless, easily startled, tearful without due reason, or tremble without due cause.

- Insomnia – getting to sleep may be difficult, sleep may be of poor quality or broken, and the patient may experience night terrors.

- An inability to concentrate.

- Memory issues compared to when the person felt more relaxed.

- Sweating, dizziness, stomach pains, heart palpitations.

- Continuous physical and/or verbal activity.

- Violence towards self or others.

Table 3.3: Symptoms of anxiety and agitation

Hermes et al., 2009; World Health Organization, 1992.

(Hermes et al., 2009). We will now undertake further discussion of mental health interventions through a consideration of processes possible under the Mental Health Act (MHA) (1983).

Using the Mental Health Act (1983) to manage risk for people with mental health issues

The MHA has significant influence on UK mental healthcare practice. The Act is divided into "sections", the majority of which deal with the administration of compulsory care. Aspects that apply to the criminal justice system are too specialist to be included here; instead, we will consider the sections used to protect people at risk of harm as a result of their mental health issues. More detail of the MHA is provided in the further reading section at the end of this chapter (p. 63).

Defining mental disorder (section 1(2))

Mental disorder is defined by the MHA as "any **disorder** or disability of the mind". Conditions commonly receiving intervention under the MHA are listed in Table 3.4. Learning disabilities and substance use need special consideration in this regard. People with learning disabilities are only covered by the Act if they display "abnormally aggressive or seriously irresponsible conduct". Addiction to substances, including alcohol, does not warrant compulsory treatment under the MHA. If a substance user experiences concurrent mental health issues, the Act may be used to treat these aspects independently.

- Mood disorders
- Schizophrenia
- Psychosis
- Anxiety disorders
- **Cognitive impairment**
- Acquired brain injury
- Personality disorders
- Disorders resulting from substance use
- Eating disorders
- Learning disabilities
- Autistic spectrum disorders
- Psychological disorders of childhood and adolescence

Table 3.4: Mental disorders most frequently covered by the Mental Health Act 1983
Department of Health, 2015.

Informal admission to psychiatric hospital (section 131)

Although much of the MHA concerns compulsory treatment, section 131 highlights that detention should be used in exceptional circumstances only. Patients should be admitted informally to a psychiatric hospital wherever safety allows. The value of admission as a means of treating the specific patient should determine the appropriateness of community or inpatient services. The potential for deprivation of liberty through hospital admission is highlighted by section 131. Accommodating informal patients on locked mental health units should be avoided whenever possible. Early intervention services should be available for patients in the community before their need becomes severe enough for inpatient admission, even as an informal patient.

Criteria for admission to psychiatric hospital for assessment (section 2)

Section 2 of the MHA allows a person to be detained in a UK psychiatric hospital for assessment and treatment for up to 28 days. They must be experiencing a mental disorder that currently places the health or safety of themselves or others at risk. The Act allows a greater degree of diagnostic doubt when utilising section 2 compared to section 3, because section 2 is used to further investigate the patient's condition. Section 2 is not renewable, and although it may be extended in exceptional circumstances, this rarely occurs in practice. Typically, a person will remain within hospital care on an informal basis or be discharged to community treatment following a lapse of this section of the MHA.

Criteria for admission to psychiatric hospital for treatment (section 3)

Section 3 of the MHA is used when a patient is experiencing a mental disorder that requires treatment within a psychiatric hospital. Treatment is seen as necessary to protect the health or safety of the person or other people. To use this section of the MHA, suitable treatment must be available to the patient, and such treatment can only be provided through detaining them using the Act. This means effective treatment is currently deemed impossible within a community setting. Section 3 applies for up to six months. This section may be removed by a mental health tribunal, or renewed by the patients' responsible medical officer if the patient continues to meet necessary criteria.

Consider the principles of the MHA covered so far when reviewing the next case study.

> ### Case study: An informal hospital admission for treatment
>
> *Matthew is a 19-year-old university student with no previous history of mental illness. Currently, he appears to be experiencing symptoms of psychosis. His parents were initially concerned by his slowed speech and bizarre ideas concerning people who Matthew feels are trying to kill him. He recently became physically aggressive towards his father when asked about these feelings, stating his belief that his father was also involved in these acts. Following this incident, Matthew was extremely remorseful, saying he wanted to die because of the thoughts in his head.*
>
> *Matthew was assessed as a matter of urgency under section 12 of the MHA. He was offered informal assessment and treatment on an inpatient unit, but refused to comply, because of fears for his own safety.*

Scenarios of the kind presented within this case study occur regularly for mental health services. A fine balance exists for practitioners between **punitive action** and allowing a person to remain at risk of potentially harming themselves or others. Activity 3.4 asks for further consideration of this situation.

> ### Activity 3.4   *Decision-making*
>
> What options are available to the mental health team assessing Matthew, and why?
>
> *A suggested answer is provided at the end of this chapter.*

Section 12 of the MHA is a key factor concerning any decision to enforce compulsory treatment in Matthew's situation.

Medical recommendations (section 12)

Section 12 of the MHA covers the process of compulsory admission to a UK psychiatric hospital. Two doctors with "special experience in the diagnosis or treatment of mental disorder" must examine the patient and agree that this person meets admission criteria under a specified section of the MHA. In most cases this will be section 2 or 3. It is preferable, but not necessary, that at least one of the doctors has previous experience in working with the patient. Up to 5 days may elapse between their examinations of the patient. Section 12 specifies that notification is given as to why the patient cannot be treated informally or as an outpatient.

Duty of the Approved Mental Health Professional (AMHP) to be satisfied that detention in a psychiatric hospital is the most appropriate course of action (section 13(2))

It is the role of an AMHP to confirm that a psychiatric hospital is the best place for treatment for the patient following a recommendation under section 12 of the Act. They are obliged to prevent admission if they view this as unnecessary or unsuitable based on "all the circumstances of the case". This may occur when a community based treatment programme is available instead of inpatient admission, and has previously helped the individual or people with similar circumstances. The views of the patient (and where appropriate their nearest relative or carers) are critical in making decisions to oppose hospitalisation under section 13(2) of the MHA.

Emergency applications for admission for assessment (section 4)

Section 4 allows compulsory admission for immediate emergency assessment to ensure patient safety. It does require a section 12 approved doctor, or a second medical opinion. Section 4 is designed as an exceptional measure when the time required to undertake an admission using section 2 of the MHA is unacceptable. This is normally due to a need to act immediately to preserve patient safety. Section 4 allows the detention of the patient in a psychiatric hospital for up to 72 hours. It is not renewable and cannot be appealed against by the patient. Following expiry of this section, the patient may remain in hospital as an informal patient, be discharged to community care or be admitted under sections 2 or 3 of the MHA.

Nurses' 6-hour holding power (section 5(4) and (5), regulations 3 and 4, and nurses order)

A registered mental health or learning disabilities nurse may detain for up to 6 hours an informal patient who is currently being treated for mental disorder in a psychiatric hospital. Detention is justifiable if the patient's mental disorder places their health or safety, or that of other people, in immediate danger. The patient may be assessed but not treated against their will during this 6-hour period. The nurse is obliged to request a medical assessment while detaining the patient. Section 5(4) of the MHA is normally used due to observed suicide risk combined with an attempt to leave the hospital setting. It should not be used merely because an informal patient is attempting to leave hospital, because unless they are at risk of harming themselves or others they retain the right to free movement.

Consider these factors while reviewing the following case study.

Case study: Attempting to leave informal hospital treatment

Emmeline is a 62-year-old woman who is being treated informally in a mental health unit. Its doors are kept unlocked except during emergencies. Emmeline becomes tearful and anxious following a telephone call from her former partner, who she recently left because of her abusive behaviour. Following this phone call, Emmeline tells hospital staff that she feels upset and wants to die. She then collects her coat from her room, stating, "I can't stand it anymore, I've got to go".

Fears for Emmeline's safety may question the wisdom of an open door policy on the mental unit described. However, freedom of movement is a right of informal patients protected by the MHA. Activity 3.5 asks for further examination of Emmeline's situation.

Activity 3.5   *Decision-making*

Imagine you are the nurse in charge of Emmeline's ward when she attempts to leave. What actions would you take, if any, and why?

A suggested answer is provided at the end of this chapter.

Central to the decision-making process required by Activity 3.5 is a consideration of the appropriateness of holding powers provided by section 5 of the MHA.

Holding power of doctor or approved clinician in charge of patient's treatment (section 5 and regulations 3 and 4)

Section 5 of the MHA allows the doctor in charge of treatment to detain a patient for assessment for up to 72 hours. Patients do not already have to be receiving treatment for mental disorder. There is no right to appeal against this section.

Medical treatment of detained patients without consent (section 63)

Section 63 of the MHA allows the treatment of patients detained by the MHA if such treatment is justifiable in their best interests. The Act specifies that "medical treatment" includes interventions to treat mental ill health by nurses, psychologists and other allied health professionals as well as by doctors. However, section 63 does not extend to all forms of treatment. Informed consent is still required for **electro convulsive therapy** and for implants to reduce male sex drive.

Warrant to search for and remove patients who are liable to be taken or returned under the Act (section 135(2))

Section 135 of the MHA allows a police officer with a warrant to enter private property to remove a person for psychiatric assessment or treatment. This is normally undertaken to recall an existing patient for treatment when their mental health has deteriorated to the extent that the health or safety of themselves or others may be in danger.

Power of police to remove mentally disordered persons from public places to places of safety (section 136)

Section 136 of the MHA provides the power for police officers to detain a person in a public place who officers believe poses danger to themselves or others due to their mental disorder. A warrant is not required for this action. Powers of detention to a place of safety under sections 135 and 136 are for a maximum of 72 hours. During this time, assessment for suitability of treatment under section 12 and 13 should take place. Places of safety include designated rooms within accident and emergency departments, psychiatric hospitals and police stations.

Leave of absence from hospital (section 17 and regulation 19)

Detained patients may be granted leave of absence from hospital by the doctor responsible for their care. Conditions of leave may be imposed for the safety of the patient or others. Typically, this involves the time period away, company kept or avoided, maintenance of medical regime and **abstinence** from substances. Periods of absence can be extended if necessary. At times, patients will only be allowed leave when escorted by a named person, usually a member of their family or hospital staff. In an emergency, section 17(4) of the MHA allows detained patients to be recalled from leave. A specific reason must be given in writing justifying this action.

Absence without leave (sections 18 and 21B and regulation 19)

Detained patients who are absent without consent from hospital, or who fail to meet conditions set within the terms of their leave under section 17 of the MHA, may be obliged to return to hospital by a police officer, member of hospital staff or person specified in writing by the hospital managers where they have been residing.

Procedure for making a Community Treatment Order (section 17A and regulation 6)

A Community Treatment Order (CTO) may be made to patients who are subject to section 3, or sections relating to criminal behaviour (sections 37, 45A, 47, 48 and 51) of the MHA. A CTO is used when the mental disorder of the patient means they require ongoing treatment to keep themselves or others safe, but such treatment remains possible outside of a hospital setting. Agreement for a CTO based upon the person's current condition and history must occur between an AMHP and the doctor responsible for the patient's care.

Recall of CTO patients to hospital (section 17E and regulation 6)

Patients living in the community with a CTO may be recalled to hospital for immediate treatment. This is the decision of the doctor in charge of their care and must be justified in terms of why they currently need to be in hospital to receive appropriate care. This is almost exclusively due to the danger posed to the health or safety of self or others resulting from their psychological condition. Circumstances prompting CTO recall normally involve a sudden deterioration in the patient's condition, often as a result of a significant life event, changes to medication regime, or substance use. Once recalled to hospital, they are subject to the same rules of treatment as other detained patients.

Duty to provide after-care services (section 117(2) and (6))

Section 117 stipulates that patients who have been subject to sections 3, 37, 45A, 47 or 48 of the MHA are eligible for after-care by mental health community services. After-care should address issues related to their mental disorder, and attempt to prevent their deterioration so that they do not return to hospital unnecessarily.

Ill-treatment of patients (section 127)

The MHA specifies mistreatment including wilful neglect of patients as a criminal offence punishable by imprisonment and an unlimited fine. Community mental health services failing to provide adequate or timely treatment for patients due to extensive waiting lists, or inpatient services that fail to provide evidence-based therapies may therefore be breaching section 127 of the MHA.

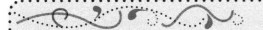

Chapter summary

Self-harm and suicide are interconnected issues that receive a great deal of input from mental health services. We know many of the factors contributing to suicide risk, but nonetheless effective assessment of individual need remains difficult. A tendency towards risk-averse

(continued)

continued . . . .

practice persists in mental health services despite the counterproductive nature of this approach. This chapter has demonstrated that health and social care professionals should concentrate on developing professional relationships with patients, because this is the most effective means of identifying individual risk and engaging service users in change. The promotion of factors protecting the individual from suicide risk is key to replacing suicide and self-harm with more effective strategies for dealing with challenging situations. The MHA supports this approach because of its emphasis where possible on non-invasive interventions, rather than using the coercive powers of the Act. Because of the potential power imbalance created by the MHA, professionals working with people with mental health issues must do as much as they can to support individuals in taking self-responsibility for their own safety. This is best achieved in community settings, using psychiatric hospital environments only when it becomes impossible to do otherwise.

Activities: brief outline answers

Activity 3.1 Critical thinking (page 45)

How you feel as a staff member following the death of one of the people you have worked with will vary depending on how much time you spend with them, the circumstances of their life, and your own personality. However, mental health teams tend to be deeply affected when patients kill themselves. Anger, guilt and regret are common reactions, sometimes with considerable blame applied to the performance of one or more team members. Suicide is almost certainly the most difficult aspect of mental health work to deal with.

Activity 3.2 Critical thinking (page 50)

The biggest risk factors here are Rubin's recent suicide attempt, which appears to be a new behaviour, his unwillingness at present to accept help through discussing what happened, and Nina's belief that he may have undisclosed financial issues. Although he is married, we have no idea of the quality of his support network. It appears that the relationship is not an entirely open and trusting one because Rubin has been unable to express himself, or Nina has not heard him.

However, we are not in a strong position to assess Rubin's safety because of the limited picture we have of him. We need to know much more about his worries, behaviour and motivations to make an effective judgement. Encouraging him to undertake a period of hospitalisation may be one way of trying to keep him safe, but may potentially be counterproductive as this takes responsibility for his own actions away from him. Spending further time with Rubin and Nina is the only clear approach to jointly assessing his needs, including suicide risk.

Activity 3.3 Critical thinking (page 53)

The mental health team is following best practice guidelines in declining Jo-Jo's admission to hospital. They are encouraging her to make use of a more appropriate service for her condition by remaining living in the community. By admitting her for treatment, the team would be furthering her belief that she cannot cope in the community, so would be disempowering her further. It is vital, however, that attempts are maintained by her community mental health worker to engage her in discussing her issues, and to work with her to find healthier alternatives to self-injury as a long-term means of remaining safe. This type of approach requires consideration, as people who habitually self-harm are at greater danger of suicide, but are best served through a community treatment approach.

Activity 3.4 Decision-making (page 57)

Matthew may be experiencing an episode of acute psychosis which is not in itself sufficient to enforce treatment under section 3 of the Mental Health Act. However, he has been violent towards another person as an apparent result of his mental disorder. He is potentially at risk of harming himself because of the intensity of his symptoms and naivety of his condition. Matthew is also unwilling to accept informal treatment. In combination, these factors justify formal assessment and treatment under section 3 of the MHA.

Activity 3.5 Decision-making (page 59)

The open door policy of this unit is entirely in keeping with the spirit of the MHA. However, the sudden change in mood and anxiety symptoms experienced by Emmeline suggest the use of section 5(4) of the MHA to allow assessment for formal treatment is justified in this case. It would be justified to lock the unit for her own protection prior to further assessment. Locking the ward without using section 5(4) would represent a deprivation of the patient's liberty so is unjustifiable.

Further reading

In-depth details of the MHA can be found in this substantial reference book:

Jones R (2011) *Mental Health Act Manual*, 14th edn. London: Sweet and Maxwell.

For rapidly accessible guidance on the MHA, see the following text:

Barcham C (2012) *The Pocketbook Guide to Mental Health Act Assessments.* Maidenhead: Open University Press.

Useful websites

Here are some of the more widely used suicide risk assessment tools. Email addresses are provided in order for readers to contact authors to request copies of the suicide risk assessment tools discussed.

Assessment of suicide and risk inventory (Black, 2013).

http://creativecommons.org/licenses/by-nc-nd/2.5/ca/tblack@cw.bc.ca

The Beck Hopelessness Scale (BHS) (Beck and Steer, 1988).

abeck@mail.med.upenn.edu

The Beck Scale for Suicide Ideation (BSS) (Beck et al., 1997).

abeck@mail.med.upenn.edu

The Columbia-Suicide Severity Rating Scale (C-SSRS) (Posner et al., 2008).

posnerk@childpsych.columbia.edu

Framework of a suicide risk assessment tool (Hawgood and De Leo, 2014).

https://www.psychology.org.au/Assets/Files/AISRAP%20protocol.pdf

The Geriatric Suicide Ideation Scale (GSIS) (Heisel and Flett, 2006).

marnin.heisel@lhsc.on.ca

The Hermes-Deakin Suicide Risk Assessment Tool (Hermes et al., 2009).

https://www.memorialmedical.com/services/behavioral-health/hermes-deakin-suicide-risk-assessment

The interRAI Severity of Self-harm (SOS Scale) (**www.interrai.org**) (Hirdes et al., 2000).

mljames@umich.edu

The Modified Scale for Suicide Ideation (SSI-M) (Miller et al., 1986).

www.gpsouth.com

The Nurses' Global Assessment of Suicide Risk (NGASR) (Cutcliffe and Barker, 2004).

cutclifi@unbc.ca

The Reasons for Living Inventory (RFL) (Linehan et al., 1983).

linehan@u.washington.edu

The SAD PERSONS Scale (Patterson et al., 1983).

brg_wmp@bellsouth.net

The Scale for Impact of Suicidality – Management, Assessment and Planning of Care (SIS-MAP) (Nelson et al., 2010).

charles.nelson@sjhc.london.on.ca

dr.amresh@gmail.com

Screening Tool for Assessing Risk of Suicide (STARS) (Hawgood and De Leo, 2015).

https://www.griffith.edu.au/__data/assets/pdf_file/0004/625846/AISRAP-Suicide-Assess-Tool-2015.pdf

The Suicidal Behaviors Questionnaire (SBQ) (Linehan, 1981).

linehan@u.washington.edu

The Suicidal Behaviors Questionnaire-Revised (SBQ-R) (Osman et al., 2001).

Suicidal Ideation Questionnaire (SIQ) (Reynolds 1987).

The Suicide Intent Scale (SIS) (Beck et al., 1974).

abeck@mail.med.upenn.edu

The Tool for Assessment of Suicide Risk (TASR) (Kutcher and Chehil, 2007).

stan.kutcher@dal.ca

Chapter 4
Mental health assessment and care planning

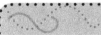

> **Chapter aims**
>
> By the end of the chapter you will be able to:
>
> - understand the theory of a nursing assessment cycle;
> - appreciate the Roper, Logan and Tierney activities of living model as a means of conducting a holistic assessment of patient need;
> - recognise the inter-related nature of each stage of an assessment, diagnosis, planning, implementation and evaluation (APIE) process.

Introduction

> **Case study: Yakiv**
>
> *Life has got too much for Yakiv. Since coming to the UK he feels troubled in his life. He finds his girlfriend difficult to live with; they have a turbulent relationship and are currently living apart. He has not been able to make as much money as he had hoped, despite working hard, and he hasn't made any real friends yet.*
>
> *Today has been particularly bad for Yakiv. He has spent all day thinking about how badly his life has turned out. He hates being alone in his flat, which is poorly insulated, so it is cold and noisy. He has been thinking about ending things. Yakiv opens his bedroom window, and thinks about jumping out. He sits on the ledge and thinks, "why not?", so he jumps.*

This case study introduces Yakiv, a person finding his life difficult. He has experienced problems which have brought him into contact with mental health services, as we shall see during this chapter. In order for the professionals working with Yakiv to be effective, they need clarity about his problems. A traditional mental health approach is to understand the patient through recognising and treating symptoms of mental illness. This is a narrow and ineffective style of service provision. This chapter describes instead a broader, holistic approach that realistically encompasses the needs of people with severe mental health issues. The key to effective mental health treatment is a well-structured cycle of assessment, treatment and evaluation. These factors are the focus of this chapter, beginning with the Roper, Logan and Tierney (RLT) model of nursing assessment.

Using the Roper, Logan and Tierney model within an APIE assessment

The purpose of the RLT model is to help the patient towards independence. The approach has similarities with Carl Rogers' theory of self-actualisation, the drive to develop fully as a human being (Rogers, 1961). RLP is an ongoing, evolving and dynamic process, rather than a "snapshot" assessment occurring when a patient is admitted to mental health services.

The RLT assessment process provides an ongoing approach to patient care. It is designed to be applied in its entirety, but in practice is often misused as a tick box exercise, focusing only on its proposed twelve activities of living. The full model is broader, considering these twelve aspects in terms of the patient's ability to undertake them independently. Using this assessment framework allows nurse and patient to develop a fuller understanding of the patient's abilities and their challenges. When utilised fully, the RLP model clarifies what the care team can do for the patient, what the patient can accomplish with help, and what they can do independently. This approach to care challenges traditional nurse–patient relationships. The RLT model encourages the nurse to adopt a coaching role where possible, recognising the patient as expert on their own health.

Activities of living are assessed in terms of current and potential independence. The RLT process must be undertaken regularly to establish how the patient is currently independent, and what they can aim towards in future. This challenging process places responsibility for change with the patient, nursing staff acting as supporters in the recovery process. It requires trust between all involved, so it takes patience, persistence and a belief in the ability of the patient to improve. Promoting independence in the patient represents recovery-focused mental health work. It contradicts traditional, psychiatrist-led, risk-averse approaches to mental health work.

The twelve activities of living suggested by RLT are:

- maintaining a safe environment
- communication
- breathing
- eating and drinking
- elimination
- washing and dressing
- controlling temperature
- mobilisation
- working and playing
- expressing sexuality
- sleeping
- death and dying.

Considering these twelve factors of individual dependence provides a comprehensive appraisal of the patient's wellbeing. Although it is often seen as a physical care model, the approach functions well within all areas of healthcare, including mental health (Roper et al., 2000).

Each of the twelve activities of living will now be discussed for people with mental health problems. This requires consideration of the following issues:

- biological factors relating to the physical health of the patient;

- psychological factors including emotions, thinking patterns and spiritual beliefs;

- socio-cultural factors referring to the impact that society and culture has upon the individual;

- environmental factors including the impact the patient's environment has on their ability to live independently, as well as the impact of the individual on their environment;

- politico-economic factors concerning the impact of governmental, political and economic aspects on the patient.

The safe environment of patients is the primary concern of most mental health practitioners. Psychologically, a patient experiencing severe emotional distress may be at considerable risk to themselves or others. This situation may lead to detention for treatment or assessment under the Mental Health Act (1983), resulting in temporary restriction of their independence. The person's socio-cultural perspective may be influential in determining need for enforced treatment. The politico-economic climate may also impact on the ability for services to provide mental health treatment, as cuts may result in services becoming unavailable. Sometimes, housing provided for people with severe mental health issues is socially isolating, compounding pre-existing physical and mental health problems.

Communication is severely limited by psychological factors for many mentally unwell people. Avoidance of others is common for people with mental health issues. Socio-cultural expectations prevent effective communication with people experiencing psychotic symptoms. Multiple environmental factors restrict effective communication for patients within mental health units. These may include the symptoms of other patients, staff with limited psychotherapeutic skills, and the perceived **hierarchical nature** of the mental health system, leading to mistrust between individuals. Politico-economic decision-making within many mental health services remains based on medical treatment rather than talking treatments, restricting opportunities to engage with patients in a psychotherapeutic fashion. Activity 4.1 provides an opportunity to consider the impact of factors highlighted by the RLT model on your ability to communicate.

Activity 4.1   *Reflection*

Many people consider freedom of communication to be a basic component of who they are. Consider the biological, psychological, socio-cultural, environmental and politico-economic factors proposed by the RLT model as factors limiting your independence in communicating. Are you surprised by what you find?

As this is a piece of personal reflection, there is no model answer.

Having considered communication as a factor influencing every human being, we now explore another fundamental aspect of existence – breathing. Breathing is significantly affected psychologically, becoming rapid and shallow through anxiety or panic symptoms. Rates of lung disease are severe for people with mental health issues, mainly due to high tobacco consumption. The perceived calming effects of smoking make it more culturally acceptable for mental health patients than for the wider population.

Many psychological issues have an impact on eating and drinking. These include avoidance of calories due to body image issues, use of food as an emotional stimulant, fears of poisoning as a paranoid world view, and eating in a ritualised fashion due to anxiety.

Biological factors include difficulty swallowing due to dry mouth or **gastro-intestinal issues**, or excessive appetite as a side-effect of psychotropic medications. It is a socio-cultural norm among mental health practitioners that significant weight gain is a necessary side-effect of antipsychotic treatment. The RLT model insists instead that nurses act to enable patients to enhance their ability to independently manage their weight, despite changing personal circumstances. Patients in a **coercive psychiatric environment**, where their right to decline medical treatment is limited, may also find independent choice of food and drink limited. Diet is not prioritised as treatment for most patients. Until this politico-economic perspective alters, food provision will remain under-resourced despite research recognising its major role in recovery from mental ill health.

Elimination can be a significant issue for mental health patients due to the constipating effects of psychiatric medication. Psychologically, anxiety conditions can make bowel movement difficult. Experiencing elimination issues of this kind may cause social withdrawal, low mood or aggression. A person with mental heath issues who perceives their environment to be threatening is less likely to spend time outside of their home, resulting in lower rates of exercise and compounding any constipation issues experienced. Politico-economic factors determine allocation of resources within mental healthcare, resulting in services often providing filling but stodgy food that worsens existing elimination issues. Where patient's access to exercise is restricted physically or through their detention under the MHA (1983), the issues described are worsened. Socio-cultural norms ensure poor bladder control remains acutely embarrassing; therefore fear of wetting oneself publicly may restrict the lifestyle of people experiencing these issues.

The ability to independently wash and dress may be affected by psychological factors. Personal hygiene may be limited for depressed individuals. Compulsive washing is common within anxiety conditions. Dress that is judged as strange may contribute to a diagnosis of mania, but this view is determined by the socio-cultural norms of the assessing psychiatrist. According to local policy, mental health patients may be required to remove belts and shoelaces when on a ward environment, regardless of their diagnosis, due to the risk these items pose to some individuals. Restriction of freedom of expression in terms of dress sense may impact on the person's self-esteem. Independent choice regarding shaving is affected when possession of sharp objects (razors) is restricted. Injury or physical health issues (such as a stroke) may reduce the ability to wash or dress independently, a factor that may be acutely embarrassing. Resulting avoidance may lead to social isolation from other patients, or confrontation with staff trying to promote cleanliness.

Controlling temperature is the factor considered in the RLT model with least apparent relevance psychologically. However, because mental and physical ill health are closely entwined, the chances of a mental health patient experiencing circulation problems is much higher than in the general population. Such problems may be compounded by cardiac issues resulting from side-effects of common psychiatric prescriptions. Poor quality insulation within rented housing will exacerbate circulatory issues, a factor that is worsened when the politico-economic environment provides inadequate housing benefit allowances, or fuel prices are high. Periods of colder weather or being located in colder parts of the country worsen these issues. Living alone is relatively more expensive, so single people may experience temperature issues to a greater extent than those in relationships.

Mobilisation often reduces when people are prescribed antipsychotic and anxiolitic medications. This represents a large proportion of people treated by mental health services. Lack of exercise is linked to low self-esteem, explaining why this commonly occurs for people with severe mental health issues. Politico-economic drivers within mental health services promote exercise as an important treatment factor, but it often remains a minor aspect of treatment compared to drug-based approaches.

Working and playing are important for recovery from mental ill health. A person who has experienced a protracted period of psychological distress may need to **re-acclimatise** themselves to interacting socially with other people. Making friends can be difficult when recent experiences have been dominated by mental ill health and its treatment. Simple interactions can be overwhelming for some people, and are significant in trapping people within the patient role. Poor physical health may limit some patients' ability to undertake some forms of work or play, but achievable alternatives are possible through effective professional–patient planning. Socio-cultural attitudes of potential employers and service users themselves may limit expectations about what types of work are possible. Breaking these **stigmatising views** is critical for reacceptance into wider society for people experiencing mental illness. Similarly, people continuing to identify themselves as patients may feel play is alien to them. The environments of many mental health units are under-stimulating, with treatment programs lacking play as a means of developing self-confidence and interaction with other people. The specific difficulties experienced by people with mental health problems in maintaining meaningful work are often overlooked by mental health treatment teams. They must instead be viewed as critical for successful recovery. The current politico-economic situation does not require people with severe mental health issues to work. This aspect may be counterproductive to recovery, because financial independence may assist psychological recovery from mental illness. Activity 4.2 seeks a consideration of work and play in your own life.

Activity 4.2   *Reflection*

How effectively do you make use of your own leisure time? Do you undertake all of the meaningful activities that you would like, or do you miss opportunities to achieve as much as you could do? If you study or work, what proportion of the time do you feel that you are achieving something worthwhile in this aspect of your life? How much of an impact do factors beyond your control have on your freedom to act as you wish to in your leisure time?

As this is a piece of personal reflection, there is no model answer.

Activity 4.2 considers independence of choice regarding work and leisure activities. Independent action may not be as available as we initially assume in these aspects of our lives, as is also the case regarding our sexuality. Expressing sexuality is an issue for many mental heath patients. Sexuality may be linked to self-esteem, and the role sexual contact has in relationships with other people. Body image is likely to be affected by previous sexual trauma, which patient self-reporting suggests is very high among mentally ill people. Frequent sexual contact may be used as an attempt to improve self-esteem for some people who have been sexually abused. Experiences of sexual exploitation are common for people who are addicted to drugs, resulting in low expectations of sexual partners and trust issues within personal relationships. Biologically, **impotence** and extreme weight gain are common side-effects from a range of psychiatric medications. These factors may limit willingness or ability to engage in sexual relationships. Misunderstanding and negative socio-cultural expectations about the nature of mental health issues may have detrimental effects when former or current patients seek to build sexual relationships with people who have not experienced mental health issues. Rates of sexually transmitted diseases may be higher than average within some social networks of psychiatric patients. These factors illustrate the extent of issues experienced by people with mental health issues concerning their sexuality.

An inability to independently control sleep patterns is a concern for many mental health patients. This can be due to anxiety or mood issues, resulting in early waking or difficulties getting to sleep. A socio-cultural norm for people with mental health problems is the use of sleeping tablets, alcohol or drugs to aid sleep. These attempts to aid sleep create severe disturbances of sleep patterns in a short time. People who are socially isolated tend to develop a sedentary lifestyle that is detrimental for sleep, rising late and consequently going to bed late.

Death and dying is a central feature for mental health patients. Distress caused by severe emotional issues urges some patients towards suicide as the only option they recognise instead of continuing with their current situation. Patients with multiple physical and mental health problems are at particular risk of suicide. Some antidepressants present paradoxical side-effects, where suicide risk is increased during early treatment. Discussion of self-harm and suicide are common between mental health patients, making it a more acceptable topic than is true for the wider population. A psychiatric environment can also increase suicide risk, as psychiatric inpatients are at particular risk of achieving suicide. Suicide rates are high amongst unemployed people and those with low incomes, aspects common for mental health patients. As well as being a major issue for people with severe mental health issues, death and dying affect every member of society, as Activity 4.3 suggests.

Activity 4.3   *Reflection*

Are you able to consider your own death? Death is an unavoidable fact of every person's life, yet we are often unwilling to accept this aspect of our existence.

What insight does considering your own death give into understanding the experience of a suicidal person, for whom thoughts of death may be an ever-present and troubling aspect of their life?

As this is a piece of personal reflection, there is no model answer.

Activity 4.3 seeks to highlight the difficulty most people have with facing troubling realities. Our professional practice will benefit significantly if we remember this when undertaking nursing assessment, a process considered in more detail next.

The nursing assessment and treatment process

Patient assessment is fundamental to all fields of nursing. The patient may be an individual, but can also be a family or group. Nursing assessment and treatment processes have been attributed to theorists including Dorothy Johnson, Ida Jean Orlando and Ernestine Wiedenbach (Yildirim and Özkahraman, 2011). Orlando is normally credited with developing the "APIE" process. This consists of assessment of patient need, planning care to reduce suffering and facilitate positive changes in health, implementation of planned changes, and evaluation as a review of care to date. APIE is a cyclical, dynamic approach to nursing focusing on the individual's needs over a period of time. It is a framework designed as an ongoing cycle of assessment that recognises that the health of the individual concerned is never static, requiring regular review and re-evaluation. The APIE nursing process is therefore appropriate to undertake patient-centred care in modern mental health work. It is this approach that we will now examine in more detail.

Assessing the patient's needs

Needs assessment involves collection of information relevant to all aspects of patient health. This is a broader approach than usually occurs in practice, where symptoms of mental and physical illness disproportionately dominate assessment processes. Effective mental health interventions are based on appreciation of patient need; as professionals, we must therefore demonstrate this understanding through recognising the multiple interlinked factors impacting on illness and wellbeing. Current and potential risk factors impacting on patient health must be identified as such, as well as appreciating personal strengths and areas for development necessary in care planning (Alfaro-LeFevre, 1999).

Assessment tools can be used to ascertain factors broadly relevant to healthy development. There are many assessment tools available, with factors investigated varying significantly between them. An assessment tool covering most mental wellbeing factors is the previously discussed RLT activities of living model of nursing (Roper et al., 2000). It presents mental health as a combination of multiple physical and psychological factors. The next case study provides an RLT assessment in mental health practice.

Case study: A holistic mental health assessment using Roper, Logan and Tierney's activities of living model

Assessment of factors determining independent living based on Roper, Logan and Tierney's model	Current capacity for independent living: *Low, Medium or High*
Patient Name: Yakiv Pshyk Date of Birth: 22/4/1975 Named Nurse: Verity Martyn Signature of person being assessed: Name and signature of person completing this assessment: Date of this assessment: 23 March 2017	
Maintaining a safe environment Yakiv is detained under section 3 of the MHA (1983) for assessment and treatment following a suspected suicide attempt involving falling from a first floor window. Yakiv is currently observed every 10 minutes due to possible suicide risk.	Low
Communication As a Ukrainian national, Yakiv has functional but not perfect English. Yakiv has limited speech, is slow to respond to questions, and does not initiate conversation.	Low
Breathing Yakiv is an ex-smoker, but has no apparent issues with breathing at present.	Full

(continued)

continued . . . .

Eating and drinking Yakiv has a BMI of 18, so he is underweight. Yakiv lacks interest in food, will eat slowly but stops eating unless continually prompted.	Low
Elimination Yakiv refuses to discuss elimination issues. He is able to attend the bathroom unaided when necessary.	High
Washing and dressing Yakiv describes self-care as "a waste of time" but will undertake it if prompted. He is able to dress himself unaided but does so slowly, due to bruising on his shoulders, abdomen and legs.	Low
Controlling temperature Yakiv reports no issues with controlling his temperature. Pulse and blood pressure are consistently within normal range.	Full
Mobilisation Yakiv is able to mobilise but is slow due to having multiple bruises.	Full
Working and playing Yakiv thinks he will have lost his job since being hospitalised. He says that he "couldn't care less" about this. At present, Yakiv declines invitations to attend social activities with other patients. He fears leaving his own room due to "other patients looking at me".	Low
Expressing sexuality Yakiv is concerned that his libido is affected by antidepressant use. He has recently split up with his long-term girlfriend.	Low
Sleeping Yakiv reports tiredness, difficulty getting to sleep and staying asleep. He is requesting sleeping tablets, as these are not currently prescribed.	Low
Death and dying Yakiv today expressed a wish to "not be here any more" but said he is "too scared" to try killing himself.	Low
Each activity of living must be considered in terms of the impact biological, psychological, socio-cultural, environmental and politico-economic factors have on the patient's ability to function independently.	

From undertaking this assessment with Yakiv, it is clear to his nurse Verity that at present he has limited independence in a range of activities of living. These issues need to be considered when they undertake the planning phase of care.

The RLT assessment illustrated in this case study provides a **holistic view** of the patient's life, rather than focusing only on their mental health. If required, an additional diagnosis-specific assessment tool may be used to record severity of psychiatric symptoms. Links to diagnosis-specific assessment tools are provided at the end of this chapter. These approaches are not broad enough to provide an effective nursing assessment of need. Symptom-specific assessment tools do not provide the information beyond severity of symptoms required to enable effective care planning. The broadness of the mental health nursing role and the narrow remit of psychiatry is highlighted by the contrasting usefulness of symptom-specific assessment tools to each profession.

Planning patient care

Following a full assessment of need, a care planning phase seeks to determine how best to eliminate suffering and improve the patient's health. Yildirim and Özkahraman (2011) suggest the factors required to plan effective care are prioritisation of need, goal setting, specifying interventions and writing a care plan. A hierarchy of issues is created based on immediate, medium and long-term need. This allows us to determine what aspects of change are necessary, in what order and how change will most effectively be undertaken. Realistic review dates may be set for each identified issue. The process breaks down complex inter-related issues into manageable individual sections, **empowering** patients to address their mental health issues.

As well as setting time scales for treating each identified health issue, responsibility must also be taken in relation to enabling required changes. For example, are planned interventions best undertaken by the nursing team, or by other health professionals? Issues occur in multi-professional teams through vacancies or sickness, or with lack of clarity of members' remit. On occasion, problems between individuals prevent work being allocated to appropriate personnel, with some staff finding delegation difficult. These factors are potential limitations to implementing care plans in some practice situations. Organisational issues of this type need to be dealt with for care delivery to become effective.

Care planning is best undertaken by setting SMART goals. This consists of ensuring objectives set are specific, measurable, achievable, realistic and time-focused. The more these factors are met when goal setting, the more likely goals are to be achieved. It is unrealistic to set goals without the direction from the patient in almost all circumstances, including severe mental illness and risk of harm to self or others. Unless the patient is entirely unable to communicate, they must be involved as fully as possible at each stage of the care process. Unrealistic care plans are developed when care staff fail to appreciate the need to plan care through the patient rather than professional perspectives. Goal setting is more effective when targeting a greater number of achievable targets than seeking fewer major achievements.

In this way patients appreciate their abilities to achieve health-related goals, creating a positive momentum for change.

Effective goals within healthcare are designed to meet individual needs. Within mental healthcare, this starts with the patient determining necessary health improvement actions. Working with them to identify relapse triggers for deteriorating mental health are critical features of goal setting. In this way, we can work with the patient to determine factors that maintain or worsen their experiences of psychological disturbance. Care planning needs to be reactive to circumstances occurring (for example, helping a person to understand their own thought processes that result in them feeling low in mood). It is also proactive in determining how positive experiences can replace negative ones. Wherever possible, patients should be given responsibility for determining necessary actions to undertake and avoid; the role of the nurse is more effective in monitoring and supporting than as a restrictive force. Of course, interventions to protect patient or public safety may be required, but this nursing role should be for as short a time as possible. In the longer term, we need to help patients develop personal health planning abilities to avoid a culture of dependency. Nurses working with patients to determine necessary health-related change should use minimal intervention in each situation to encourage their independence beyond the psychiatric system. Care planning, wherever possible, must be patient-led.

The planning stage culminates with the creation of a care plan document. The format for doing so varies across practice areas, the main focus being its usefulness to staff and patient. Care plans fail when they are formulated from the perspective of professionals rather than patients. To be useful, they are the property of the patient and should be accessible throughout care. Care plans must be dynamic, evolving documents that demonstrate the transparent mental healthcare between patient and staff. It guides decisions during care interactions and must cover all aspects of treatment currently planned with the patient. This approach entirely opposes **generic** or pre-determined care plan documents. These generalised plans are a barrier to self-determined healthcare, representing the most unimaginative and ineffective healthcare provision. Conversely, effective care plans are always individualised, creative in their approach to care and are developed whenever necessary to fit the patient's changing needs.

Having considered the main aspects of care planning, we can now consider the RLT process undertaken between Yakiv Pshyk and Verity Martyn.

Activity 4.4	*Planning care based on findings from an assessment of need using Roper, Logan and Tierney's activities of living model*

Review the factors identified by Yakiv and Verity in the previous case study (see p. 73). Using SMART principles, develop suitable actions and determine their priority as a means of completing this partially completed care plan. An example of how necessary actions might be developed is provided at the end of this chapter.

Care plan following an assessment of need based on Roper, Logan and Tierney's activities of living model	Priority for action:
Patient Name: Yakiv Pshyk	*None, Low, Medium or High*
Date of Birth: 22/4/1975	
Named Nurse: Verity Martyn	
Signature of person receiving care:	
Name and signature of person completing this care plan:	
Date of this care plan: 23 March 2017	
Date evaluation of care is due: 30 March 2017	
Maintaining a safe environment Moving towards independent personal safety is critical for Yakiv following his recent suicide attempt. *Action*:	
Communication Yakiv's lack of pro-active communication may be a symptom of low mood. *Action*:	
Breathing	None
Eating and drinking Yakiv's current lack of interest in food may be a symptom of low mood. *Action*:	
Elimination A possible side-effect of Yakiv's new medication is gastro-intestinal upset and difficulty urinating. *Action*:	
Washing and dressing Yakiv's lack of self-care may be a symptom of depression. *Action*:	
Controlling temperature	None
Mobilisation	None
Working and playing Yakiv's lack of social interaction and interest in the future may be symptoms of low mood. *Action*:	

(continued)

continued . . . .

Expressing sexuality Yakiv's reported sexual dysfunction may be a significant self-esteem issue and a potential reason for discontinuation of medication following future discharge from hospital. *Action:*	
Sleeping Yakiv's sleep disturbance may be a cause of his low mood and is also a symptom of depression. *Action:*	
Death and dying Yakiv has expressed suicidal thoughts but also fears of dying. *Action:*	

Activity 4.4 provides an opportunity to develop a comprehensive and easily monitored care plan based on the previous assessment made by Verity with Yakiv. Because of his current circumstances, his identified needs are likely to require medium or high priority for action. For each point, emphasis should be placed on Yakiv in leading changes as much as possible himself, rather than relying on care staff to make decisions for him. Although he currently has a highly dependant role, particularly in terms of maintaining his own environment and communicating with others, the unified purpose of his care plan is to enable independence as fully as possible in the optimum time necessary. The plan must be specific in its aims, as well as the tasks required of Yakiv and the healthcare team. This makes it simple to review in terms of outcomes met and changes needed during the evaluation phase of the APIE process, allowing an effective understanding of what has worked and what needs to be changed within Yakiv's next APIE cycle.

As Activity 4.4 demonstrates, assisting the patient as fully as possible in planning their own care is a skilled business that can take a considerable amount of trust and time. In some instances this could be on a scale of several years and during multiple periods of treatment. It is an approach that is often unappreciated by mental health staff, but one that we need to embrace in order to become as effective as possible in enabling mental wellbeing and reducing the incidence of mental ill health. Having determined as fully as possible with the patient a set of SMART care aims, we need to work with them on implementing these factors within practice.

The implementation of planned care

If a substantial and effective process of assessing need and planning care has taken place, the process of **implementation** becomes relatively straightforward. If assessment has not been conducted thoroughly and effectively, or if necessary planning processes are limited or flawed, the process of implementation is hugely limited. It is true that planned care is often actualised in different and surprising formats than originally proposed; however, this eventuality becomes much more likely when assessment and planning protocols have not been followed adequately. A skilled and experienced mental health practitioner may be able to undertake effective interventions on an ad hoc basis, but sustained improvement is made much more achievable when a strong pattern of intention stretches between all four areas of the nursing assessment process.

Although implementation warrants a section in its own right, its enactment should be considered directly when planning interventions. Where the planning process identifies the nature of interventions and who will deliver them, the question of exactly how they are delivered is a matter for implementation. The greater the degree of precision applied to each intervention (for example, why and when it will be delivered, for how long, and alternatives if it becomes unfeasible or is declined by the patient), the more direction can be applied to the nursing process. After all, it is the ability for interventions to facilitate change or prevent decline in the patient's health that is central to the evaluation process. Having considered implementation of planned care, it is necessary now to consider its evaluation.

Evaluation of care

The recording of interventions undertaken is usually included as a task within the planning section of the APIE model. On consideration, it is more realistically described as an **evaluation** rather than intervention aspect of the process, because any intervention undertaken should be followed by an immediate informal evaluation of effectiveness. Within mental health nursing practice, this function can take the format of case notes for the patient. Where possible, best practice involves the patient themselves being involved in writing up of session notes. This is important because it allows them to own the process of evaluation, rather than being a passive participant in this aspect of their own care. Taking self-responsibility of this kind is a fundamental aspect of becoming mentally healthy.

Reporting progress made, as well as any difficulties experienced when undertaking planned interventions, directly links the implementation and evaluation phases of care. It allows more immediate changes to be developed between the patient, individual practitioners and the multidisciplinary care team than is possible through utilising formal evaluation sessions alone. Reporting processes are set during the planning phase. Changes to planned care must be made with due consideration for outcome improvement, but failing to update processes when they are proving to be ineffective suggests a rigidity to planning protocol that is likely to be seen as unnecessarily authoritarian by the patient.

In order to undertake a formal evaluation of care in an effective manner, the following questions need to be asked regarding the patient's care plan: Which outcomes set have been achieved at this point? How effective were each of the interventions used to achieve these outcomes? Which interventions should be continued, altered or removed from the plan? What changes, if any, now need to be made to the plan of care to optimise its effectiveness?

Following this assessment of the effectiveness of the current care plan, a reassessment of the patient's needs at this moment is made. New or ongoing objectives of care are planned, implemented and evaluated in a cycle that continues until the patient's health issues are resolved, or they withdraw from the care process. It is likely to take multiple APIE cycles to optimise care for the individual patient. The nature of severe mental health issues is that they can be intense, complex and long-standing. A much greater reliance by service personnel on the evaluation process of care is necessary to optimise treatment provided for patients with severe and enduring mental health issues. Currently care tends to be provided in an episodic fashion – instead, we need to link periods of care and good health together in a much more formal fashion to inform our assessment of individual patients' needs. In this way, our ability to plan and implement care with them becomes much more effective. The case study below provides an evaluation of care that links assessment, planning and implementation together as pre-emption to another cycle of assessment.

Case study: An evaluation of care based on a care plan using Roper, Logan and Tierney's activities of living model

Patient Name: Yakiv Pshyk	*Result of this review of care: None, Low, Medium or High priority for patient and care team as an action for independence*
Date of Birth: 22/4/1975	
Named Nurse: Verity Martyn	
Signature of person reviewing their own care:	
Name and signature of person completing this evaluation of care:	
Date of this evaluation of care: 30 March 2017	
Date of reassessment/review: 7 April 2017	
Maintaining a safe environment	Yakiv said today that he agrees with the care team's view that maintaining a safe environment should remain a **high priority for team action** as it significantly impacts on his ability to live independently.
Action: Yakiv's detention under the MHA (1983) and regular observation are under weekly review by his care team. Yakiv has asked for these aspects to be reviewed and the care team agree to remove both of these factors as soon as it appears safe to do so.	
Achievement of action: Following a review (7 April 2017) by the multi-disciplinary team, Yakiv remains detained under section 3 of the Mental Health Act, but has been deemed safe today to require informal observation only. This is due to his reported increase in mood over the last week, supported by Yakiv's viewpoint and team observation of apparent reduced symptoms of depression compared to those at the time of his admission for treatment.	
Effectiveness of interventions: Through the process of undertaking observations every ten minutes, the care team has provided regular opportunities for Yakiv to speak with them about his concerns. During these conversations Yakiv has expressed an awareness on 6 April 2017 that this period of treatment has been a necessary means of protecting him from hurting himself following his recent suicide attempt.	

Sustainability and format of interventions: Yakiv no longer needs to be observed formally, but his status as a detained patient will remain under weekly multi-disciplinary team (MDT) review. He has agreed to continue spending an hour each day in therapeutic conversation with a member of his care team (see "Death and Dying").	
Communication *Achievement of action:* Yakiv says that he now trusts the healthcare team more and knows that they are trying to help him. He agrees with staff observations that he is now able to communicate in a much freer style. His case notes record that he has been observed to be initiating conversation with staff and other service users on multiple occasions every day for the last week. This is viewed by staff as one indicator of an increase in his mood. Yakiv says that he thinks this is "probably true". He states that he is "a quiet person" but was "much less talkative than normal when I first came to hospital". *Effectiveness of interventions:* The care team agree with Yakiv that this intervention has achieved its objective as he is now able to talk in a much more open manner. *Sustainability and format of interventions:* Yakiv recognises that he no longer needs formal monitoring of his communication, but has asked staff to remain aware that if he becomes less willing to speak this is a sign that he is anxious.	Because of his recent improvements, Yakiv's ability to independently communicate is a **low priority for current action**.
Breathing No action is required currently.	
Eating and drinking *Achievement of action:* This intervention has been partially successful so far, as Yakiv agrees with the observations of the care team that he is showing more independence in eating, but that his BMI of 19 means that he remains underweight. Yakiv has set a target of returning to 60 kg; this represents a healthy BMI of 24. He has asked to make this increase "naturally, in my own time" so does not wish to set a timescale for doing so. *Effectiveness of interventions:* The style of intervention seems to be successful, as Yakiv is making progress towards a safer weight, having increased BMI from 18 to 19 since admission. *Sustainability and format of interventions:* Yakiv no longer warrants such direct encouragement to regain independence regarding	Yakiv's eating and drinking currently warrant **low priority for team action**.

(continued)

continued . . . . •

eating. He says that he feels confident to attend the dining room for meals with other patients and believes he is capable to undertake his own decisions regarding food. He has agreed to being weighed weekly as a means of monitoring his continued progress towards regaining a healthy weight. This will take place as part of Yakiv's review of care.	
Elimination *Achievement of action*: As Yakiv is in a period of transition between his previous medication and a new prescription, monitoring of elimination continues to be relevant due to potential side-effects. Yakiv is completing daily elimination charts with prompting from the care team; he says that he recognises the purpose of doing so. *Effectiveness of interventions*: To date, issues with elimination have not been apparent. *Sustainability and format of interventions*: This action is relevant to Yakiv's newly prescribed antidepressant, so monitoring should continue on a daily basis until medication is fully titrated into his system. The care team is following manufacturer's recommendations that this is likely to take another two weeks.	The possibility of side-effects mean this intervention remains of **medium priority for action** by Yakiv and the care team to help him regain independence.
Washing and dressing *Achievement of action*: In order to undertake necessary self-care, Yakiv currently receives twice daily prompting to wash, dress and clean his teeth. *Effectiveness of interventions*: This intervention has not yet resulted in independent action by Yakiv. *Sustainability and format of interventions*: The care team feel that this is a suitable format for intervention that may require more time to lead to independence; Yakiv declines to comment on this aspect of his care, despite being asked for his viewpoint.	Yakiv's washing and dressing remain a **medium priority for action** for the healthcare team to help him regain independence.
Controlling temperature No action is required currently.	
Mobilisation No action is required currently.	
Working and playing *Achievement of action*: Yakiv continues to require significant prompting to attend patient groups but has done so on a daily basis during the last week. He has once (29 March 2017 at 14:15)	Yakiv and the care team agree that working and playing remain a

opted to spend time socialising with other patients without prompting, but today reports being "anxious" about doing so. *Effectiveness of interventions:* Yakiv today said that he has difficulty spending time in the company of other people, but doing so will help him "become more confident". This suggests that the intervention is working to some degree but is not yet complete. *Sustainability and format of interventions:* Yakiv acknowledges that this intervention is "useful" and he needs "more practice to benefit from it". He says that he is willing to attend therapeutic groups provided on a daily basis, and to spend an hour each evening with other patients in social activities after dinner. Yakiv recognises that staff prompting him to do so may be necessary.	**medium priority for action** to help him regain independence.
Expressing sexuality *Achievement of action:* Yakiv has been prescribed a different antidepressant anticipated to have less impact on his libido than his previous medication. Yakiv reports that he is yet to appreciate the result of this change because the transition between drugs has not yet fully taken place. Yakiv says he is glad that he has been able to express his feelings in writing to his former girlfriend. *Effectiveness of interventions:* Yakiv said today that he appreciates that his sexuality has been taken seriously regarding this change in antidepressant medication. The effectiveness of the change of prescription is yet to be determined in terms of the impact of the new drug on Yakiv's libido. *Sustainability and format of interventions:* Yakiv and care team are in agreement that ongoing monitoring of this side-effect is very important because of its impact on Yakiv's ability to act independently. Yakiv has asked for private discussion of this aspect of his care with his doctor during weekly medication reviews.	Yakiv's ability to express his sexuality remains of **high concern for action** by his care team to help him regain independence.
Sleeping *Achievement of action:* Yakiv has undertaken changes suggested by the care team to his sleeping pattern, achieved following prompting on most days. *Effectiveness of interventions:* Yakiv reports that this intervention has been partially successful in improving his sleep. *Sustainability and format of interventions:* Yakiv says the approach is "helpful" but he does not "always feel like" making necessary	Because of the partial progress made by Yakiv, his independent sleeping is now a **medium priority for action** by the care team.

(continued)

continued . . . .

changes. Yakiv suggests that the format should remain unchanged at present, with him going to bed to read at 10 p.m. and attending breakfast at 8 a.m. He suggests that prompting to undertake both actions is realistically necessary for him at present.	
Death and dying *Achievement of action:* The goal of Yakiv meeting members of the healthcare team for one hour daily to discuss the situation leading to his suicide attempt has been achieved to date. *Effectiveness of interventions:* Yakiv said today that this process has been "very helpful" in enabling him to understand his motives for jumping from a window, in developing his confidence in speaking to others about issues, and recognising some possibilities for a more positive future. *Sustainability and format of interventions:* Yakiv and the care team are in agreement that this intervention remains useful in its present format of daily private conversations for an hour with one of his designated nurses.	Independence concerning death and dying remains a **high priority for action** by Yakiv's care team to help him regain independence.

For this evaluation of care, the following factors should be considered:

Was each outcome achieved?

How effective were the interventions used?

Should each outcome be continued, altered or removed?

What changes to the care plan or new objectives are now required?

The case study above demonstrates the uneven nature of progress when working with a person experiencing symptoms of severe mental ill health. Yakiv can be seen to be making significant progress in some aspects of his life, but has developed little in others during the short period of inpatient treatment covered. Having undertaken a review of the theoretical and practical aspects of the APIE nursing assessment and treatment process, it is now possible to consider the assessment process in more detail through examining the work of Roper, Logan and Tierney (2000).

The examples covered in this chapter consider some of the many issues experienced by people with mental health problems that impact on their ability to undertake independent living activities. Through applying the model in its full form, the RLT model can be seen to provide a good framework for a holistic assessment of factors affecting the quality of life of people using mental health services. However, it lacks a specific focus on relationships as an important factor within the formation and treatment of mental health problems. This is an illustration of why an assessment model of this kind is insufficient alone when seeking to understand issues presented by a patient. Instead of a complete process, it represents a useful prompt for more advanced decision-making skills based on individual interaction. Any assessment model remains insufficient without the use of effective interpersonal communication between those involved.

The RLT model of assessment provides an opportunity to identify and treat in combination the physical health issues experienced by most people with severe mental health problems that have traditionally been overlooked by many services. In practice, activities that nurses feel uncomfortable discussing are often ignored. This leads to assumptions by the wider care team that the patient does not have issues in this area, when in fact they haven't been allowed to discuss the subject. For effective practice, healthcare teams need to ensure that each member is utilising their chosen format of assessment in an acceptable and realistic fashion.

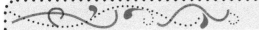

Chapter summary

We have considered in detail Yakiv's experience in working with a mental health treatment team, with specific examples of the assessment, planning and evaluation phases of his treatment. The RLT model has been utilised in conjunction with the APIE model of nursing care. These processes illustrate the need to undertake a much broader consideration of holistic care than is traditionally the case within mental health services. In order to be effective, treatment approaches need to develop sufficiently to encompass the multi-faceted reality of mental health issues, rather than retaining an inappropriately narrow symptom-specific focus. Fundamental to this is the developing definition of the mental health nurse's role to become one that meets the real needs of the modern mental health patient.

Activities: brief outline answers

Activity 4.4 (page 76)

Care plan following an assessment of need based on Roper, Logan and Tierney's activities of living model	Priority for action:
Maintaining a safe environment *Action*: The care team will review Yakiv's detention and ten minute observations on a weekly basis, with the aim of removing these factors as soon as it is safe to do so. Safety is indicated by a reduction to an acceptable level of symptoms of low mood, social withdrawal and suicidal ideas.	High

(Continued)

(Continued)

Communication Yakiv has limited speech, is slow to respond to questions, and does not initiate conversation. *Action*: Members of the care team will actively encourage Yakiv to talk to them as a central aspect of his inpatient treatment. This can occur as part of his ten minute observation process, and also on an individual basis every day for up to an hour with a designated member of the care team.	High
Eating and drinking Yakiv's lack of interest in food may be a symptom of low mood. *Action*: Because Yakiv is underweight, the nursing team should negotiate a healthy target weight with him. The team can encourage Yakiv to eat a standard portion of food at mealtime and monitor his BMI until he regains a normal appetite.	High
Elimination *Action*: Because Yakiv has refused to discuss elimination issues, it may be useful to explain to him more effectively why taking his prescribed medication makes monitoring of his elimination necessary. By gaining his cooperation, the care team will be able to ask Yakiv if he is experiencing any elimination problems on a daily basis, and if necessary amend his medication accordingly.	Medium
Washing and dressing *Action*: Yakiv's self-care (washing, dressing, oral hygiene) will be encouraged morning and night by care staff.	Medium
Working and playing *Action*: The nursing team will encourage Yakiv to attend patient therapeutic groups every morning, and social activities every evening. Yakiv has agreed to spend at least one hour of social time with other patients on the unit every evening; nursing staff will remind him of this at 8 p.m. each day.	Medium
Expressing sexuality *Action*: Because sexual dysfunction is a common reason for discontinuation of medication, Yakiv's prescription should be reviewed as soon as possible by his medical team. Options for alternative treatment could be discussed with Yakiv to find an approach that is acceptable to him. If changes to medicines are made, monitoring of this side-effect will need to occur for at least the titration period; this may take several weeks.	High
Sleeping *Action*: Developing a daily sleep and exercise programme acceptable to Yakiv may help him to relax. Staff may prompt Yakiv in going to bed and rising at suitable times (for example, 10:30 p.m. and 8 a.m.). Yakiv may be better avoiding strenuous exercise until his injuries have healed; this aspect can be reviewed weekly and begun at a suitable time.	High
Death and dying *Action*: If Yakiv is willing to do so, allocated members of the care team could spend one hour daily with Yakiv in an individual structured therapeutic fashion, discussing the situation that led to his suicide attempt.	High

Further reading and useful websites

The Beck Depression Inventory II (BDI-ii) is available at:

https://static1.squarespace.com/static/5205b3d1e4b08b89e5d18f2a/t/520ae965e4b0bc18c970b0f0/1376446821340/Beck-Depression-Inventory-and-Scoring-Key1.pdf

The BDI-ii is the most widely used depression-specific paper assessment tool, so is useful to be familiar with in order to appreciate its usage in diagnosing mood disorders.

An alternative assessment tool to the BDI-ii is the Patient Health Questionnaire (PHQ-9), available at:

http://www.cqaimh.org/pdf/tool_phq9.pdf

Like any document of this type, the PHQ-9 should be used only to indicate that a further assessment needs to take place, rather than as a definite diagnosis.

The Beck Anxiety Inventory (BAI) is available at:

http://www.brandeis.edu/roybal/docs/BAI_website_PDF.pdf

Although not as familiar as the BDI-ii, BAI is often used by practitioners as a means of screening for common mental health disorders.

Chapter 5
Psychotherapeutic approaches to mental healthcare

> ### NMC Standards for Pre-registration Nursing Education
>
> This chapter will address the following competencies:
>
> **Domain 2: Communication and interpersonal skills**
> 1. All nurses must build partnerships and therapeutic relationships through safe, effective and non-discriminatory communication. They must take account of individual differences, capabilities and needs.
> 2. All nurses must use a range of communication skills and technologies to support person-centred care and enhance quality and safety. They must ensure people receive all the information they need in a language and manner that allows them to make informed choices and share decision-making. They must recognise when language interpretation or other communication support is needed and know how to obtain it.
>
> **Domain 3: Nursing practice and decision-making**
> 3.1 Mental health nurses must be able to apply their knowledge and skills in a range of evidence-based individual and group psychological and psychosocial interventions, to carry out systematic needs assessments, develop case formulations and negotiate goals.

> ### NMC Essential Skills Clusters
>
> This chapter will address the following ESC:
>
> **Cluster: Care, compassion and communication**
> 7. Consistently shows ability to communicate safely and effectively with people providing guidance for others.
> 8. Communicates effectively and sensitively in different settings, using a range of methods and skills.
> 11. Is proactive and creative in enhancing communication and understanding.
> 12. Uses the skills of active listening, questioning, paraphrasing and reflection to support a therapeutic intervention.

Chapter aims

By the end of the chapter you will be able to:

- understand the basic principles of four major forms of **psychotherapy**, and explain these to relevant interested patients and colleagues;
- recognise and explain to patients the presence of unhealthy behaviours, emotions and thought patterns;
- apply new knowledge of therapy processes when undertaking patient referrals for specialist therapeutic input;
- begin to apply core therapeutic techniques in your practice work with patients.

Introduction

Case study: Poor communication skills

One of the saddest events I have witnessed occurred when I was working in an elderly care ward. I was working as a cleaner in the summer holidays before starting my nursing course at university. Every day I spoke with the more communicative patients. One afternoon, a nurse wheeled an elderly gentleman from the TV room to his bed area, drawing the curtains around him. I heard her say to him, "I have some bad news, your wife has died. I'm going to leave you for a while now so you can be alone." The nurse then opened his curtains and left the area. The patient was sobbing.

I was shocked by the way in which this news had been given and the lack of comfort given to this man when he was in such need. I told the man how sorry I was; he held my hand and said, "She was my wife." Even with no experience of healthcare, I felt this episode was an appalling avoidance of care from nursing staff towards a person in great need of comfort.

This situation illustrates a lack of compassion and effective communication skills that are core requirements of nursing practice. This chapter examines core theory underpinning the psychotherapeutic approaches most commonly used in modern healthcare in an attempt to address these communication skill deficits. We examine techniques used to improve communication with people experiencing emotional and psychological difficulties. These skills are presented in a straightforward manner to aid understanding for those who may not be entirely familiar with this aspect of healthcare.

Appropriate caution is needed when any new skill is practised with the public. This applies to the psychotherapeutic approaches covered in this chapter. Clinical supervision from an experienced colleague is therefore recommended to ensure safe and effective practice takes place.

The techniques presented in this chapter should therefore be undertaken with personal competence in mind, and under supervision from a suitably qualified practitioner.

We begin by considering the aims and process of psychotherapy, followed by examining the relevant features of the **psychodynamic**, person-centred, **cognitive** behavioural, and brief solution-focused approaches. The skills featured are under-represented across all fields of nursing, having as much relevance in adult and children's nursing as mental health work. Particular focus is made on informing readers about relevant practical skills in each area covered.

The aims of therapy

The aims of therapy vary between the different approaches, and according to individual therapists' interpretation; however, a common set of aims can be summarised as:

1. Facilitating emotional and psychological development.
2. Reducing the impact of traumatic life events through planning and enacting necessary changes.

The therapy process

Rather than one approach, psychotherapy includes a range of theories for understanding the self and other people. It is primarily used to heal psychological issues, but also has enormous benefits in developing good health of well-adjusted individuals. Hundreds of variations of psychotherapy exist; to cover all of them is unnecessary here, so the most commonly used approaches have been selected for further examination.

Psychodynamic therapies

The work of Sigmund Freud and further developments by later psychodynamic therapists was the start of modern psychotherapy. It emphasises the impact of parental figures and childhood experiences as principal factors in developing our adult personality, expectations and behaviour. Consequently, the psychodynamic approach focuses on early experiences as the source of psychological and emotional disturbances persisting in the present. Psychodynamic theory is traditionally expert-led, specialist in application, and diagnostic in explaining mental health problems. The most useful aspects of the approach therefore need adapting for use by non-specialist health professionals in situations such as John's.

Case study: John

Farouk is a Child and Adolescent Mental Health Services (CAMHS) staff nurse. He is asked to work with John, a 12-year-old boy referred for help with anger issues. On meeting John, it is clear to Farouk that his anger issues are specific to his family home. There are no reports of problematic behaviour at

---

school, and he answers questions calmly when Farouk meets him individually. He is consistent in his view that his mum often speaks to him angrily, and this causes arguments. Farouk met with Joanne, John's mum, to discuss the situation; she became tearful when explaining that her parents had alcohol problems, and although they loved her they were distant when she was growing up. Joanne felt her own parenting has influenced her relationship with John, as she finds showing affection towards him difficult. Joanne explained that she often shouts at John because she doesn't feel she can cope as well as she should; however, she wants to learn to relax and teach him not be so angry. Joanne tells Farouk that Steve, her partner of eighteen months, gets on well with John and is much more able to demonstrate affection for him.

Farouk met with John, Joanne and Steve to discuss the situation. At an emotional meeting, the adults listened to John's concerns. They agreed to work on speaking calmly with each other rather than shouting. They met again the following week and then the following month; the family reported a situation that wasn't perfect but was much improved. Steve had mediated between Joanne and John on one or two occasions, but the biggest change had been in Joanne becoming more comfortable in demonstrating affection to her son, rather than being jealous or irritated by him.

This situation is an example of weakened attachments between mother and child. Arguably, early life experiences have impacted on Joanne's adult life. By reflecting on our childhood experiences, we may understand the person we have become as an adult. In examining psychodynamic therapy, you may wish to consider how these ideas relate to your own **family dynamic**.

Psychodynamic therapy introduces the concepts of the unconscious mind and conflicting internal drives. An awareness of these concepts may help us to recognise why changes necessary to achieve a healthy lifestyle are so difficult to undertake. The relative strength of the conscious compared to the unconscious aspects of the mind determines how we act. Our patients may experience inner conflict between conscious and unconscious emotional drives, consciously understanding the need to make difficult changes while unconsciously denying the probability of a threatening health condition. We only need to think of patients diagnosed with cancer who continue to smoke to see these processes in action.

Psychodynamic theory suggests our parental figures (including family friends, siblings, grandparents, aunts and uncles, as well as parents themselves) are hugely influential in the development of our personalities. This is because children unconsciously copy the behaviours they see displayed. The health promotion process must therefore emphasise that parental health choices significantly influence their family unit. For example, a coronary patient successfully undertaking a weight reduction programme will provide significant additional health benefits for their children, partner and wider family through sharing healthier meals together. More importantly, the patient's children will learn useful life skills by seeing their parent taking responsibility for their improved health.

Psychodynamic therapy provides the theory of ego defence mechanisms, the best known examples being denial and rationalisation (Corey, 2009). These mechanisms underpin irrational human behaviour as an attempt to protect the ego from threatening stimuli. An awareness of ego defence mechanisms can explain why people behave in a frustrating, counter-productive fashion. By raising this awareness, we may help them to understand and moderate their behaviour in a healthier way. To be effective, focus must be on exploring issues together rather than overtly challenging the service user. As a collaborative process, the service user is supported to address difficult issues raised. An explanation and example of each ego defence mechanisms follows.

Ego defence mechanisms in practice

Ego defence mechanism	Characteristics of the ego defence process	Examples of ego defence mechanisms in practice
Repression	Repression keeps thoughts or memories that threaten the ego away from conscious awareness. These repressed thoughts remain unconsciously influential of our behaviour and emotional reactions. The unconscious influence of repressed material may be demonstrated through slips of the tongue, dreams, or lapses of memory that reveal hidden motivations.	*Aggressive or sexual dreams reveal unfulfilled animal instincts; mistakes in language express unconscious desires (saying "sex" instead of "six", for example).*
Denial	Denial involves blocking from conscious awareness aspects of life that we find too threatening to deal with. For the person experiencing denial, it is as though the threatening stimuli don't exist.	*Smokers are able to continue smoking through not admitting the negative impact this behaviour has on their health.*
Projection	Projection involves believing my feelings towards another person are actually the way they feel about me. This justifies feeling persecuted or hostile towards them. Projection blames other people for our own socially unacceptable impulses, and negates responsibility for our own feelings and actions.	*I hate them, so I believe they hate me. The way I believe they feel about me allows me to hate them back – I am defending myself rather than attacking them.*
Displacement	Displacement attempts to satisfy socially unacceptable impulses through other means. Unsatisfied impulses are directed onto a powerless target or symbolic substitute, as the real target is too threatening.	*Displacing anger towards my boss through instead shouting at my children.*

Regression	Regression is the adoption of childhood behaviours as an adult during times of stress. This is an attempt to recreate safety feelings experienced as a child through the hope of invoking care, attention, or special allowances from others.	*Eating chocolate when stressed, or having tantrums when overwhelmed by stressful situations.*
Sublimation	Sublimation satisfies socially unacceptable impulses through creative expression. This is often viewed as a constructive defence mechanism, but avoids the causes of troubling issues.	*Aggression is often taken out through sport; anxiety is directed into art or music; suffering and art seem to exist together.*
Projective identification (introjection)	Unconsciously adopting the characteristics, opinions or behaviours of another person who exerts a powerful emotional influence. These ways of being may contradict our key values, creating internal emotional conflict.	*Bullied people commonly mirror the bullying they received themselves, despite feeling this way of behaving is unreasonable.*
Rationalisation	Events are distorted by rationalisation to make them less threatening. Reasons are invented to justify unpleasant behaviour, failures, or weaknesses of the self or others.	*A person rationalising their mistreatment of their partner may say: "I only get angry with you because I love you."*
Reaction formation	Hiding feared thoughts and feelings from others and ourselves through behaving in the opposite way to our real feelings.	*People displaying homophobic behaviour may actually have homosexual drives they wish to hide and fear to express.*
Conversion anxiety (somatisation)	The expression of emotional pain as physical symptoms.	*Muscular tension (particularly backache), head and stomach-aches occurring at times of stress.*
Compensation	Rather than dealing with personal deficiencies in functioning, the person develops other areas in their life instead.	*A person may develop their money-making potential in an attempt to feel happy rather than dealing with their difficulties in relating to other people.*
Disassociation	Feeling of not really being present, like an actor in a film, or really being someone else.	*Troops in combat roles and people experiencing physical or sexual assault report this experience.*
Acting out	Extreme physical behaviour as a means of expressing thoughts and feelings that the person feels unable to verbalise.	*Suicide attempts, physical violence to others, destroying inanimate objects, drug use.*

Defence mechanisms are varied and complex; their further exploration is requested in Activity 5.1.

Activity 5.1   *Reflection*

Having reviewed the theory of ego defence mechanisms, it is likely that some of these ideas particularly resonate with you, and others make no sense at all. Think about the ego defence mechanisms you tend to adopt in threatening situations, and those that you rarely seem to use. Make a note of your thoughts now, then review them after you are next in an emotionally charged situation. Do you actually only use the ego defence mechanisms you originally suggested in these situations?

As this activity is based on your own observations, there is no outline answer.

Having considered ego defence mechanisms as core aspects of psychodynamic theory, we now consider a radically different alternative in the person-centred approach.

The person-centred approach

Carl Rogers developed his counselling theory as a radical alternative to psychodynamic therapy. Rogers' person-centred approach (PCA) emphasises the self-responsibility of the client for creating and therefore changing their own life. It highlights that people with whom we work are experts on their own situation. This alters the role of health professionals from experts on what is best for the patient, to a resource for clients to consult when making health decisions. In adopting this approach, care professionals need to recognise that the decisions clients make may not necessarily be what we hope for. With these factors in mind, consider the next case study.

Case study: Mrs Tsang

Cath is a staff nurse working on a busy medical-surgical unit. One of the patients in her care, Mrs Tsang, has been recovering from an operation after breaking her hip. During her hospital stay, Cath has observed symptoms of dementia in Mrs Tsang. This suggests she may be unsafe if she returns to her existing living situation.

Mrs Tsang is visited regularly by her daughter Sue, who is her long-term informal carer. Cath wishes to gain a fuller understanding of Mrs Tsang's social situation as part of an ongoing assessment of her needs. Cath uses the person-centred approach as the basis for her communication with Sue and Mrs Tsang on her next visit. This allows Sue and Mrs Tsang to explore the pros and cons of returning to her own home, and the alternative of residential care. Cath chose this communication approach because she has previously seen nursing staff unduly influencing families, with decisions which the relatives later regretted. Mrs Tsang and Sue are given time to consider available options,

---

with Cath helping them answer these difficult questions. Through this process, Mrs Tsang decided that additional support would be helpful to enable her to remain in her own home. Sue thanked Cath for supporting her in having this discussion with her mother, as previously she had refused to admit to needing help. Sue emphasised the benefit of being listened to through Cath's approach, rather than receiving advice on what to do.

This situation describes an adult nurse letting go of her expert role in advising on health choices. It requires an investment of time by allowing a patient to plan her own health. By rejecting an expert-led approach, PCA develops communication between equals. Topics for discussion are therefore determined by the client, not the professional. This approach seems counterintuitive to nurses who believe their professional role is to advise patients on health decisions. However, being trusted by professionals to make their own decisions ultimately allows clients to make most progress in counselling.

PCA theory suggests client-led change is the only way to achieve effective psychological, emotional and behavioural developments. Central to the approach are Carl Rogers' *necessary and sufficient conditions for personality change.* This requires the counsellor to be congruent (honesty in expressing their own thoughts and feelings), empathic (accepting the client's feelings about their experiences even when this contradicts their own viewpoint), and unconditional in positive regard towards the client (appreciating their worth as a person, regardless of their views and behaviour). We cannot reject clients because we find them unpleasant, or be friends with them because of the one-way nature of counselling dialogue. The client and counsellor have to be in psychological contact, this being the willingness to work together in examining difficult issues. Rogers believes all clients fluctuate in their ability to be fully honest about themselves and their experiences; it is useful to remember this when working with a client struggling to express themselves honestly (Rogers, 1957).

The PCA is strictly non-diagnostic in its interpretation of mental health problems. It views the diagnostic system within psychiatry as damaging vulnerable individuals it seeks to treat. Categorising individuals according to symptoms of mental illness is limited in practice because it does not focus on positive change. Rather than this focusing on personal deficits, the PCA facilitates the client to make necessary changes a reality.

Where the psychodynamic approach focuses on the past, PCA is focused on present events. Rather than concern with troubling past experiences, the PCA asks how past events relate exclusively to present circumstances. Although past events are highly influential on present perspectives, we can't change our past. We can instead minimise the impact of past events on our present and future life. The PCA emphasises every person's ability to make changes, recognising this may be a radically new perspective for some people.

The development of most communication skills can be found within the PCA. Here are definitions, purposes and examples of these techniques.

Communication skills in practice: practical therapeutic techniques

C: Client   P: Professional

Techniques	Definition	Purpose	Example
Reflection (McLeod and McLeod, 2011).	Using the clients' own words by repeating their meaning back to them as accurately as possible.	Allowing the speaker to expand on their own thoughts, and demonstrating the value of exploring their chosen topic further.	C: "I don't want to live any more." P: "You don't want to live any more."
Paraphrasing (Evans, 2007).	Restating, in different words, the views expressed by the client.	Paraphrasing checks the precise meaning of statements made, demonstrating the professional's understanding, and encouraging more detail.	C: "I want to kill myself." P: "You feel like dying?"
Summarising (Evans, 2007).	Stating in the briefest form the main themes expressed by the client over a substantial period of the session.	Demonstrates the listener accepts and recalls the client's views over a period of time. It may also be used to restart conversation following a period of silence.	P: "So far, you have talked about your relationship with your sister, how you worry about money, and your marriage. Which of these do you want to discuss next?"
Open questions (Evans, 2007).	These questions require an expansive answer, rather than a "yes" or "no" response.	Open questions encourage more detail on the client's perspective, allowing them to continue discussing their chosen subject.	[at the start of a session] P: "What do you want to talk about today?"
Closed questions (Evans, 2007).	Questions that require a definite answer.	Closed questions ensure answers on specific issues. This is useful when the client has avoided answering previous questions.	P: "Have you ever asked them why they do this?"
Synthesis (Simmons and Griffiths, 2009).	Relating specific information provided to other relevant topics already raised during therapy.	This allows connections to be made between broad themes the client may not have recognised previously.	P: "How do these problems with alcohol relate to the relationship issues you previously talked about?"

Downward arrow technique (Thomas and Drake, 2012).	Retaining focus on each issue raised by the client, pursuing answers for further detail on each topic.	This approach expands discussion of a single topic, developing understanding of issues raised.	C: "I'm feeling depressed." P: "What do you mean by depressed?" C: "I mean I don't enjoy my life." P: "What don't you enjoy about your life?" C: "I don't like the way my kids talk to me." P: "What is it about the way they speak to you that you don't like?"
Challenge (Evans, 2007).	Pointing out contradictions between statements apparent when considered in the context of each other. Also, asking for evidence for strongly held views when little evidence has been provided to support them.	Highlighting the incompatibility of contradictory opinions makes changes of perspective inevitable.	C: "I can't do it." P: "Why can't you do it?" C: "Because I couldn't do it last time." P: "Yes, you couldn't do it before. But why does that mean you can't do it now?" C: "I don't know; I suppose it's just because I haven't tried."
Disclosure (Corey, 2009).	The professional deliberately reveals an aspect of their own life that is relevant to issues raised by the client.	This process helps the professional clear their mind of obtrusive thoughts, improving their concentration on the client's dialogue. It is also useful for the professional to role model an ability to experience difficulties without deteriorating into crisis.	C: "I have a problem appreciating anything good about myself." P: "I have difficulty feeling good about myself too." C: "Really? You always seem so together." P: "It helps me to share this with you; I'm doing my best to like myself more."

(Continued)

(Continued)

Immediacy (McLeod and McLeod, 2011).	This is the professional stating how they feel about the things the client has discussed, or the interaction taking place between them.	Immediacy emphasises the impact therapeutic work has on the professional as well as the client, humanising the counselling relationship.	**P**: "I am finding what you are talking about upsetting because it seems to have been so hard for you to deal with."
Modelling (Corey, 2009).	Modelling involves the client recognising others demonstrating more effective ways of dealing with situations the client struggles with.	Modelling proves changes the client views as impossible can be achieved given changes in their approach.	**P**: "Who do you know who copes better with confrontation than you?" **C**: "My boss – he never seems to get angry even when people are rude to him." **P**: "So, what do you need to do to be more like your boss when you experience conflict?"
Use of silence (McLeod and McLeod, 2011).	Allowing the client longer to consider their thoughts than is usual in everyday conversation. This emphasises the benefit of considering fully the topic being discussed.	Therapeutic silence gives the client time to gather and express their thoughts; it values their need to think more than the professional's need to talk.	**C**: "I'm not sure what to say now." **P**: "That's ok, take your time." [Silence] **C**: "It's good to clear my head. Can we look at what we talked about earlier again now?"

Consider the PCA communication skills we have reviewed when undertaking Activity 5.2.

Activity 5.2   *Communication*

During interviews for nurse education courses, most candidates claim to have strong communication skills. The NMC (2010) recognises communication as a skill essential for effective practice, yet poor communication is responsible for most of the failings identified by the Francis Report (2013). With this in mind, review the PCA communication skills. Which of these skills are you already aware of, which do you use in practice, and which don't you use but have seen being used by colleagues? You may then identify which of these skills need more practice, and which you need to use for the first time. Spending time with colleagues competent in these areas would be very useful for your own professional development.

As this activity is based on your own observations, an outline answer is not available.

Having reviewed your own application of PCA skills, the next approach to consider is cognitive behaviour therapy (CBT) because it utilises so many of these skills directly.

Cognitive behaviour therapy

CBT can be described as a set of approaches, rather than a single theory of therapy. This is confusing because textbooks and individual practitioners vary considerably in their interpretation of CBT. For this reason, practical features common across CBT approaches are highlighted in this chapter, rather than discussing the technical differences between CBT formats.

CBT theory does not challenge the diagnostic categorisations of mental illness. It is often used in conjunction with the prescription of psychiatric medications. This accounts in part for CBT being the therapeutic approach of choice within psychiatric settings. More research supports the use of CBT compared with other styles of psychotherapy. However, we should view this evidence cautiously as research undertaken considers many different versions of CBT, making results difficult to compare with each other.

CBT theory emphasises the relationship between thinking, emotional and behavioural processes. This is seen as causing and maintaining all psychological disturbance; reduction of troubling experiences is seen as the clients' responsibility. This contrasts with the commonly held view that upsetting emotions result from external circumstances. CBT suggests instead that the way we interpret events is what disturbs us, rather than events themselves. Our reactions to difficult situations do not necessarily have to result in our suffering.

An innovation brought by CBT is linking of work between sessions through therapeutic tasks. Although some textbooks refer to this process as homework, this term is best avoided because of potential negative connotations. Therapeutic tasks can take any useful format through negotiation led by the client. A thought diary is a common therapeutic task covering the client's thoughts during stressful, pleasurable and neutral situations over a week.

A major role of CBT is educating clients about the role of psychological processes in creating and maintaining psychological distress. This psycho-educational function is often the main feature of CBT group work. Group and individual CBT processes are different but similarly informed treatments. Understanding this is important when making referrals for specialist CBT in order to appreciate what treatment is actually offered to patients.

Cognitive errors are unrealistic ways of thinking that allow thoughts that lack evidence to become believable. These common ways of thinking provide immediate explanations during stressful situations. They simplify challenging issues because they do not take into account the wider context or the full range of evidence occurring within relevant situations. Our role as health professionals is to help our patients to identify when they are making cognitive errors, and to help them to replace these irrational thinking patterns with more realistic evidence-based thoughts. Here are examples of each of Beck's (1973) cognitive errors, with rational counter explanations.

Cognitive errors

Type of cognitive error	Explanation of the unhelpful, un-evidenced cognitive error process	Example of the cognitive error and a rational alternative
Arbitrary inference	Taking only a limited amount of available evidence and drawing significant conclusions from it.	Error: "I know I won't be able to do it because I couldn't before." Rational alternative: "I found it difficult previously but this doesn't make it impossible."
Personalisation	Feeling personally responsible for events beyond our control.	Error: "If I was a better parent my son wouldn't always be so unhappy." Rational alternative: "I admit my imperfections as a parent, but my son has his own opportunities to improve his life as an adult."
Depersonalisation	Not taking responsibility for our own actions or inactivity.	Error: "Of course I hit him, he made me angry." Rational alternative: "I chose to hit him when I was angry, I had alternatives but didn't think about them."
Minimisation	Under-estimating the importance of an event or circumstance.	Error: "What's the problem, it's only a few drinks." Rational alternative: "Drinking isn't a problem in itself, but my behaviour when drunk can be."

Maximisation	Over-estimating the importance of an event or circumstance.	Error: "I didn't get into Cambridge, my life is completely ruined." Rational alternative: "I really wanted to get into Cambridge and I am upset about not doing so, but I can still enjoy studying elsewhere."
Polarisation	Holding a viewpoint that a person, object or event is either all good or all bad.	Error: "I love everything about her." Rational alternative: "I love her, even though she has faults like everyone else." Error: "I can't stand being near him." Rational alternative: "I find these aspects difficult about him . . . ."
Cognitive filters	Taking notice of only the good (positive filter) or the bad (negative filter) in a situation. Albert Ellis believes people tend to wear either "Rose coloured glasses" or "Shit stained spectacles" (Ellis, 1962).	Error: "When we have a baby everything will be perfect." Rational alternative: "I am looking forward to having a baby, but at times there will still be issues to deal with in my life." Error: "I'm old and useless, I can't do anything any more." Rational alternative: "I have to make realistic allowances for my physical limitations because of my age, but there are still many things I can do."
Awfulisation (Dryden and Yankura, 1993) Catastrophising (Beck et al., 1979)	Holding an unrealistic view of the level of distress (awfulness) associated with a situation.	Error: "This is the worst possible thing that has ever happened to me." Rational alternative: "This is very hard to deal with; I will need to persevere to get through it." Error: "I won't ever get over this." Rational alternative: "It is going to take time to come to terms with this event."

As well as an identification of cognitive errors, schema theory is central to CBT. Schemas are rigid, and therefore unhelpful, patterns of thinking or beliefs about past, present and future events. They are based on personal perceptions of past experiences, and exclude present circumstances. Problematic **schemas** apply to Beck's "Cognitive Triad" of the self, others and the world.

The schema model of consciousness

Level of cognition	Description	Example
Conscious awareness	Deliberate, focused current attention applied to a personally specified area of interest.	"I'm currently thinking about what to write now as an example of conscious awareness."
Pre-conscious awareness	Automatic thoughts – whatever we are thinking at any particular time, occurring without personal direction.	"I'm hungry." "This is boring."
Simple schemas	Our individualised way of doing things which occur without thinking.	The way we walk, write, open doors, our accent.
Intermediate beliefs	Rules and assumptions about ourselves, other people, and the future. They are characterised by the use of *should, must, can't* statements, and "*If . . . then . . .*" and "Yes, but . . ." statements.	"I *should* be happy." "They *can't* be trusted." "Things will *never* change." "*If I* trust anyone *then* they will let me down." "I am angry because I can't do anything about it." "You should be earning more money at your age." "If I wasn't fat then I would be happy." "Yes I should exercise, but I'm always too busy."
Core beliefs	Rigid simple beliefs about ourselves, other people, and the future.	"*I am* stupid." "*Other people* can't be trusted." "*The world is* a threatening place."

Thought record sheets are used to record issues, potential solutions and progress undertaken through CBT. They cover the main aspects of the CBT process. Because there is no set format, the simple version presented in Figure 5.1 is open to development according to the needs of individual patients and health professionals.

Keep the factors covered in terms of cognitive errors and schemas in mind when undertaking Activity 5.3.

A. Activating Event, if known (*Trigger*)				
B. Irrational, un-evidenced and unhelpful Beliefs about *Activating Events* (*A*)				
C. Consequences of these unhelpful Beliefs (*B*)				
Emotions	Thoughts	Behaviour	Physical	Social
D. Disputing Beliefs (rational, evidenced, helpful beliefs disputing section *B*)				
E. Evidence for and against the original Beliefs (*B*)				
E. Evidence for and against the new Disputing Beliefs (*D*)				
F. Finding Out (*Behavioural Experiment – evidence supporting both B and D*)				
G. Goals (*Moving focus away from problems towards alternative ways of being*)				

Figure 5.1: Thought record sheet

Source: adapted from Ellis (1962).

Activity 5.3   *Reflective practice*

The most effective way of understanding how other people think is to explore our own cognitive processes. One method of doing so is by addressing a troubling issue within your own life through completing a thought record sheet. This can be anything of concern from your professional or personal experience. Undertaking this exercise will take some time and effort, but it should help you to understand yourself better, as well as developing your understanding of CBT. It will also provide insight into the emotionally demanding requirements of being a client experiencing CBT.

As this activity is based on your own observations, an outline answer is not available. However, a completed thought record sheet is provided at the end of the chapter as an example, and can be used in comparison to your own document.

The thought record sheet can be seen to be one of the major developments of modern therapeutic practice. Another introduced by CBT is the behavioural experiment. They are practical activities developed by the patient. They gather evidence for and against troubling beliefs and their rational alternatives. They can be undertaken by the patient alone, or with a health professional as the feared experience is deliberately encountered. This is termed "in vivo" working and is a form of graded exposure (see p. 105). Behavioural experiments aim to help the patient to move from a stuck or avoidant position to one of greater psychological freedom. This occurs by gathering evidence that contradicts their former irrational position, and strengthens their belief in rational alternatives.

The communication skills developed within the person-centred approach should be fully utilised within CBT practice. However, additional CBT specific skills also exist. Examples are listed here.

CBT specific communication skills

Techniques	Definition	Purpose	Example
Live (in vivo) working (Neenan and Dryden, 2004).	Deliberately creating a problematic scenario with a client in order to support them in re-engaging with the avoided situation, and allowing a discussion of the issue as it occurs.	Live working increases the effectiveness of treatment by dealing with an issue as it manifests, rather than losing accuracy by discussing it after the event.	An **agoraphobic** person could go shopping with a health professional, discussing their thoughts, feelings and actions as they occur.
Behavioural experiments (Neenan and Dryden, 2004).	Behavioural experiments are activities planned to test evidence for the unhealthy and alternative beliefs that have been highlighted in therapy.	Behavioural experiments create real life evidence that supports the belief that significant change is actually possible.	Someone who fears flying would need to take a flight to test their rigid belief that they will be too panicked to manage it.
Flooding (Dobson, 2001).	Deliberate full exposure of the client to a feared situation or stimulus, with or without the professional present.	By exposing the client to the feared stimulus, it is demonstrated to be unpleasant rather than actively harmful to the client.	A person who is scared of drowning could be encouraged to dive into a swimming pool (with appropriate safety precautions).

Graded exposure (Simmons and Griffiths, 2009).	Gradual progressive exposure to a feared situation, with or without the professional present.	Graded exposure is based on a belief that sudden exposure through flooding can itself be traumatising and therefore counterproductive.	For a person with a snake **phobia**: graded exposure could involve progression from talking about snakes, to looking at pictures of snakes, visiting a zoo and holding a snake.

Having reviewed CBT, it is apparent that it provides a comprehensive explanation of psychological cause and effect. This contrasts with the approach undertaken by brief solution-focused therapy (BSFT), the next approach for consideration.

Brief solution-focused therapy

Rather than considering how mental health issues are caused, BSFT helps clients to find realistic means of enabling change to take place. It is probably the easiest psychotherapeutic approach to use, with potential for great benefit from participants. An example of the approach is given in the next case study.

Case study: Simon

Simon was admitted to A&E following an overdose of paracetamol. Many staff in the department feel frustrated with him because of the self-inflicted nature of his action; they have also been critical of the assessing psychiatrist in not admitting him for mental health treatment. David, an A&E staff nurse, recognises that the NMC Code of Practice (2015) suggests more should be done to help this patient. Being aware that he may not see Simon again, David uses communication based on BSFT. He asks Simon directly what he wants to be different about his life; had his overdose achieved this change; and what could Simon do to make necessary changes happen. Simon struggled to answer these questions, prompting David to re-ask each question several times. Because of this, Simon identified that speaking honestly with his family about his situation might help him get the help he needs. With encouragement from David, Simon phoned his father. He told him he had taken an overdose, and arranged to spend time staying with his parents. David's role did not allow him to monitor Simon's progress over time; however, Simon hasn't been admitted again due to further overdose, suggesting he is making positive changes in his life.

This case study demonstrates the power of simple, challenging questions asked repeatedly when a person feels their troubles are intractable. BSFT moves away from professional-led change through emphasising self-responsibility and ability for health improvement within every person.

It aims to refocus the client away from their problems, instead emphasising the benefit of seeking solutions for issues experienced. The clients' concerns are accepted, but the approach seeks movement away from a position of **learned helplessness** or "stuckness" in problem situations. BSFT highlights the ability of individuals to cause, and therefore solve, their emotional issues. This is often underappreciated by those experiencing the issues themselves.

Each session of BSFT is undertaken independently, rather than being part of a wider pattern of therapy. This is because clients may not return for further therapy. The approach therefore seeks to maximise impact of each session at the time it occurs, rather than assuming further meetings will take place. This attitude reflects the reality of much healthcare work, as many individuals in greatest need attend appointments sporadically.

BSFT is a non-diagnostic approach, as it does not use diagnostic categories of mental health problems. It also does not present a theory of mind, since it does not explain why psychological issues exist. For some patients and health professionals this is hugely empowering; for others, it is unnerving and nonsensical. Despite these omissions, BSFT is nevertheless able to create effective psychotherapeutic change through focusing on meeting the needs of each individual service user. This is achieved through a series of techniques developed within BSFT, including solution focused questions, scaling, reframing and rolling with resistance.

Solution-focused questions (McLeod and McLeod, 2011) are central to BSFT technique. They are used to deliberately focus the client on what they wish to achieve, and what they will do to get there. In this way, they help the person to move on from a negative focus on perceived problems, so are particularly useful when feelings of being stuck predominate. Causes of issues experienced are never denied, but focusing on them is not seen as productive because doing so does not lead to solutions. What is important instead are questions that address the person's aims, and the objectives that will make this aim attainable. BSFT questions therefore include: "What does the person want to experience?"; "What must happen for this situation to occur?"; "What can you do to achieve it?" These are direct but supportive questions that may have to be asked several times in order to receive a considered answer.

Scaling (Simmons and Griffiths, 2009) involves asking the client to describe where they see their situation on a scale of 1 to 10. Here, 1 represents the worst situation possible, and 10 represents the best it could be. Scaling is often used poorly, as numbers alone are of no use without putting them in context. Scaling should only be undertaken to help the client plan how they may move from their current score to a more favourable one. For example, "If your situation is currently a 3 out of 10, what would have to happen to make it 4 out of 10?" Once the person has answered this question, it would be appropriate to ask "What would make it a 10 out of 10 situation?" Working towards a realistic solution in this way is a useful means of developing an achievable target for personal development.

By placing a new frame on a familiar painting we change the image from worn out to fresh. Thus, the term reframing is a means of changing a view of a familiar problem. The reality of the picture (or problem) does not change, but its appearance does, mainly because we now look at it more. The reframing process is a "skeleton key" that has potential to help in any situation regardless of presenting issues (Thomas and Drake, 2012). It encourages a shift from negative to realistic thinking by considering circumstances in their entirety. For example, Kevin is a person with alcohol issues who has recently become intoxicated. Kevin perceives this as a failure because he wishes he didn't drink anymore. However, viewed objectively this situation is broader than Kevin's evaluation. A realistic evaluation of his situation recognises that Kevin has succeeded in not drinking for six days this week. He has therefore succeeded much more than he has failed. People tend to recognise negative experiences much more readily than positive ones. This means positive aspects of events are easily overlooked. The reframing process first involves accepting the impact the issue has on the client. Accepting these negative realities makes it difficult for the client to deny the professional's presentation of positive realities also occurring in their situation. Reframing therefore presents previously unconsidered aspects of a situation, rather than allowing negative viewpoints to go unchallenged. To maximise learning in Kevin's situation, it would be appropriate to ask, "How have you succeeded in not drinking for 6 out of 7 days?" in order to help him replicate his successful behaviour.

Rolling with resistance (Miller and Rollnick, 2002) is a useful approach in conjunction with reframing. The approach involves the health professional agreeing with the client when they claim they are incapable of influencing their situation. Agreement is surprising as people often seek to deny negativity in others as a means of reassuring them. By supporting the clients' negative view, a paradoxical effect often occurs, with the client arguing against their own inability to facilitate change. The client's resistive energy is channelled into a recognition of the possibilities for change. An example of rolling with resistance occurs in the next case study.

Case study: Rolling with resistance

C: *Client*   **P**: *Professional*

C: *"It doesn't matter what anyone says – I know I am no good at anything."*

P: *"I agree – you are useless at everything."*

C: *"Well I'm not rubbish at everything – just things like speaking with people I don't know very well."*

P: *"I agree – you seem shy rather than totally useless."*

Having reviewed a range of communication techniques presented by BSFT, this knowledge is required in the next activity.

Activity 5.4   *Team working*

Within teamwork situations, issues may occur where individuals clash because of different worldviews. Consider an area of conflict occurring in your own practice experience. What solution-focused questions would you ask in this situation, and what options would you predict to develop as a result?

As this activity is based on personal observations, an outline answer is not available at the end of this chapter.

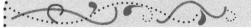

Chapter summary

This chapter has addressed the key aspects of the major branches of modern psycho-therapy. It has considered the communication techniques required to put psychotherapy theory into practice across all fields of healthcare. Practitioners in all areas will benefit from using these approaches when working with patients, families or peers experiencing any form of emotional or psychological issue. The best way to develop communication skills is to put these techniques into practice through integration with our current work, and reviewing developments through critical reflection with our trusted colleagues.

Activities: brief outline answers

Activity 5.3 An example of a completed thought record sheet (page 103)

Thought record sheet, adapted from Ellis (1962/1990)

A. Activating Event, if known (*Trigger*)
Being shouted at by my teacher in infants' school when I was five, as I was blamed for someone else having knocked over a vase of water.

B. Irrational, un-evidenced and unhelpful Beliefs about *Activating Events* (*A*)
1. *I'm not going to try because things will go wrong* (this was initially regarding education, but later extended to other creative activities).
2. *Other people can't be trusted* (as whoever knocked the vase over let me take the blame for it; and the teacher used her position of power to intimidate me).

C. Consequences of these *unhelpful Beliefs* (*B*)

Emotions	Thoughts	Behaviour	Physical	Social
Anger. Feeling insecure.	Other people have treated me badly, so they will do it again. I mustn't be vulnerable ever again.	I avoid starting activities that are new to me.	Shortness of breath during verbal confrontations, even when of little genuine consequence.	Bearing grudges against people who upset me.

D. Disputing Beliefs (rational, evidenced, helpful beliefs that dispute **B**)
1. *If I try something new and things go wrong, this doesn't have to automatically impact on the way I feel. I am not as good at things the first time as after I practise them, so it's fine not to be good initially.*
2. *People can be trusted, but to different degrees. I am secure in discovering how much this is the case for each individual through spending time with them. This allows me to approach others positively until I have reason to do otherwise. It also allows me to accept that other people may not meet my own level of trustworthiness without this unduly upsetting me.*

E. Evidence for and against the original Beliefs

1. *I'm not going to try because things will go wrong* (this was initially regarding education, but later extended to other creative activities).

For: Some things have and will continue to go wrong in my life on a daily basis. These are never pleasing occurrences. This feels unfair.

Against: Just because things go wrong doesn't mean I have to be deeply upset by them. I can't even think of anything that has gone seriously wrong in recently times. My experience of life doesn't seem fair or unfair, it is the way it is.

2. *Other people can't be trusted* (as whoever knocked the vase over let me take the blame for it; and the teacher used her position of power to intimidate me).

For: Some people I have met are not worthy of trust with personal information or are uninterested in helping other people.

Against: I don't have to put any faith in other people's willingness to help me out; when I most need it people will be there or they won't be, there is nothing I can do about the nature of other people.

E. Evidence for and against the new Disputing Beliefs

1. *If I try something new and things go wrong, this doesn't have to automatically impact on the way I feel. I am not as good at things the first time as after I practise them, so it's fine not to be good initially.*

For: Over the last few years I have become experienced in pushing myself outside of my comfort zone as a means of experiencing new things and learning new skills (learning a language, doing DIY, moving to new parts of the country).

Against: Sometimes I will feel disheartened by the size of the challenges I face and failures I experience in undertaking new things. This, however, I know is perfectly normal.

2. *People can be trusted, but to different degrees. I am secure in discovering how much this is the case for each individual through spending time with them. This allows me to approach others positively until I have reason to do otherwise. It also allows me to accept that other people may not meet my own level of trustworthiness without this unduly upsetting me.*

For: When I experienced serious issues at work some years ago, the people I thought I could rely on were of little help, and some of those who I knew less well proved to be much more supportive than I had expected them to be.

Against: I want the people I associate with to be entirely trustworthy regardless of circumstances, but this is unrealistic so is not going to be the case in reality.

F. Finding Out (*Behavioural Experiment – evidence supporting both B and D*)

1. *Testing the impact of failure on myself*

I will record my own thoughts, emotions and behaviour when experiencing failure. This could be undertaken through deliberately attempting an overly advanced activity – for example a challenging set of physical exercise or advanced language class.

2. *Testing the trustworthiness of other people and its impact on me*

I will deliberately open up to the people I suspect are least trustworthy in my current social environment to see if they prove to be as untrustworthy as I imagine, and also to test the impact this has on my thoughts, feelings and behaviour.

G. Goals (*Moving focus away from problems towards alternative ways of being*)

Having undertaken this exercise, I am keen to develop further my acceptance of the fallibility of both other people and myself.

> I would like to become more emotionally self-sufficient and less reliant on the support of other people to feel positive about myself and my life.
>
> By achieving this, I aim to become more forgiving of other people when they are selfish or misguided without being unrealistically positive about their motivations.

Further reading and useful website

The books written by Windy Dryden are particularly accessible to practitioners, being written by a therapist with practice in mind. He covers all forms of CBT and provides practical examples of approaches described. A useful starting place is *Be Your Own CBT Therapist: Teach Yourself* (2011) published by Hodder and Stoughton, or *Cognitive Behaviour Therapies* (2012) published by Sage.

Gerald Corey writes about the forms of psychotherapy covered in this chapter as well as other important approaches. His writing is easily understood and is valuable for those interested in developing their therapeutic skills. *Theory and Practice of Counselling and Psychotherapy* (2009) published by Brooks and Cole is an ideal general textbook on psychotherapy.

The *In a Nutshell* series of books from Sage publishers cover the different forms of psychotherapy in a succinct manner – these are ideal texts for those learning about the approaches for the first time. For example, *Rational Emotive Behaviour Therapy in a Nutshell* (2005) by Michael Neenan and Windy Dryden covers the original form of CBT in a simple but informative fashion.

Carl Rogers' books (particularly *On Becoming a Person*, 1961) are often recommended as core texts within therapy education. However, they are theory heavy rather than practice focused. This contrasts with the films made of his counselling work, which are easily accessible. *Three Approaches to Psychotherapy* (1965) directed by Everett Shostrom is a film featuring Carl Rogers in practice, and is particularly valuable as a guide to healthcare staff wishing to develop their empathic skills. A link to the film is available on YouTube: **https://www.youtube.com/watch?v=SgiX0QLnpBM**

Chapter 6
Psychopharmacology

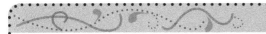
Chapter aims

By the end of the chapter you will be able to:

- describe the majority of drugs prescribed within modern psychiatric treatment;
- acknowledge which medications are recommended for each psychiatric condition;
- appreciate the pre-existing physical health conditions experienced by patients that make the use of each drug potentially dangerous;
- identify potential side-effects resulting from the use of each medicine described.

Introduction

> ### Case study: Kareem
>
> *Kareem is a patient with a diagnosis of schizophrenia being treated in a psychiatric admission ward under section 3 of the Mental Health Act (1983). He is angry about this deprivation of his liberty, remaining in his room and refusing to respond to staff questions regarding his welfare. Several years ago he was prescribed fluphenazine, an intramuscular antipsychotic injection. It is therefore suggested at a multi-disciplinary meeting that he is again treated with this drug. Attempts are made by staff to explain this decision to him, and to seek his informed consent for treatment with this drug. As Kareem refuses to accept this form of treatment willingly, he is informed by staff that the Mental Health Act (1983) allows them to administer this medicine even against his will. It is argued by his prescribing doctor that his unwillingness to accept prescribed treatment is the result of his mental illness. Kareem accepts his medication peacefully, but states that he is only doing so because he feels that he has no other choice.*

The actions taken in enforcing Kareem's medication are legal, but are far from ideal. Taking treatment decisions away from the patient is potentially damaging for the therapeutic relationship between staff and patient. In Kareem's scenario, he is assumed to be incapable of making a reasonable decision because of his psychiatric diagnosis. This assumption is not necessarily correct, as the Mental Capacity Act (2005) highlights that patients held for treatment under the Mental Health Act (1983) may retain capacity for decision-making. Staff providing Kareem's care make their decision without acknowledging all relevant legislation, and fail to discuss fluphenazine's side-effects with him. Kareem is therefore not given sufficient information to understand the implications of this treatment. Without appreciating potential side-effects, early awareness of their presence may be missed. This is dangerous when being treated with such a potentially hazardous medicine.

Despite major advances in availability of non-pharmacological options, medication remains the primary treatment for most people experiencing psychiatric symptoms. This is surprising considering the insufficiency of evidence supporting the effectiveness of psychiatric medication, and because of the non-toxic alternative of evidence-based psychotherapy. When considering range and severity of side-effects present with psychotropic medicines, it is concerning that patients are willing to take them, and practitioners remain prepared to dispense them. This may be due to a lack of appreciation of the physical health risks these substances pose. The *British National Formulary* (BNF) (2016) is the primary reference guide to medications currently licensed for use in the UK. Other drugs are prescribed elsewhere in the world, but are not regarded as safe in UK medical practice, therefore are beyond the scope of this book. The BNF lists the disorders suitable for treatment by each drug, the physical health conditions experienced by patients that make a medicine unsafe, and the side-effects caused by each drug. This last factor is of prime importance for any professional involved in the care of people with mental health problems. In order to support service users in their choices concerning psychiatric medication, we must be aware of the potential health costs of using these substances.

Traditionally, mental health education focuses on the physiological processes of medicine. In practice, this is of little use when advising patients about the reality of treatment. What matters instead is the impact each medicine is likely to have on the physical health of the person taking it. The primary focus of this chapter is therefore on the side-effects inherent in each group of medicines commonly used in psychiatric practice. By appreciating these risks, we are able to meet our ethical obligation to provide our patients with necessary information to make informed choices about their use of psychiatric medications.

This chapter considers medicines that are termed antipsychotic, hypnotics, anxiolytics, drugs used for the treatment of mania and hypomania, and antidepressant medications. For each category of medicine, we will consider the conditions they are recommended to treat. The main focus of the chapter, however, is the impact of potential side-effects on patients receiving them. We begin by considering antipsychotic medications as the primary treatment for psychosis, followed by medication for insomnia, anxiety, mania and depression.

Antipsychotic medication

Case study: Sean

Sean is a young man experiencing symptoms of psychosis for the first time in his life. He is supported closely by his family, allowing him to remain living in his own home. He has been prescribed risperidone, reporting side-effects of breast enlargement and loss of sex drive. Sean asks his psychiatrist for a change of treatment, but is urged to persevere with his current medication in order to prevent deterioration in his condition.

Soon afterwards, Sean's parents begin to suspect that he has not been taking his medicine. When they confront him, Sean walks out and is missing for several days, being picked up by police in a disturbed state of mind. Sean is admitted for treatment to a psychiatric unit under section 3 of the Mental Health Act (1983), where he is prescribed various psychotropic medications with limited effect.

The situation experienced by Sean presents little empathy for his views as a patient. Alternatives to risperidone are not explored, and Sean's concerns for his physical health are given inadequate consideration. Admission to hospital is a serious event, and may have been avoided here if Sean's views were appropriately considered. Too often the assumed psychological benefits of psychotropic medications are given absolute priority regardless of the side-effects experienced by the patient. Giving Sean greater responsibility in decision-making may have resulted in a better outcome for him than the period of hospitalisation described.

Antipsychotics are categorised as two distinct generations of drugs. They are often referred to in practice as neuroleptics or major tranquillisers. This latter term accurately describes their physical, psychological and emotional numbing effects. The older forms of antipsychotics are listed in Table 6.1.

Original drug name	Alternative names	Recommended as treatment for:
Benperidol	Anquil	Deviant antisocial sexual behaviour
Chlorpromazine hydrochloride	Chlorpromazine Largactil	Schizophrenia and other psychoses Mania Short-term management of psychomotor agitation, violence or dangerous impulsivity Anxiety/agitation
Flupentixol	Flupenthixol Depixol Fluanxol	Schizophrenia and other psychoses Depressive illness Not suitable for symptoms of mania or psychomotor hyperactivity
Haloperidol	Dozic Haldol Serenace	Schizophrenia and other psychoses Mania and hypomania Short-term management of psychomotor agitation, violence or dangerous impulsivity Anxiety/agitation
Levomepromazine	Nozinan	Schizophrenia
Pericyazine	Periciazine	Schizophrenia and other psychoses Short-term management of severe anxiety, psychomotor agitation, violence or dangerous impulsivity Anxiety/agitation
Perphenazine	Fentazin	Schizophrenia and other psychoses Psychomotor agitation, violence or dangerous impulsivity Short-term management of anxiety Mania Anxiety/agitation
Pimozide	Orap	Schizophrenia and other psychoses

Prochlorperazine	Buccastem Stemetil	Schizophrenia and other psychoses Mania Short-term management of anxiety
Sulpiride	Dolmatil Sulpor	Schizophrenia
Trifluoperazine	Stelazine	Schizophrenia and other psychoses Short-term management of psychomotor agitation, violence or dangerous impulsivity Anxiety/agitation
Zuclopenthixol	Clopixol	Schizophrenia and other psychoses
Zuclopenthixol acetate	Clopixol Acuphase	Short-term management of psychosis and mania

Table 6.1: First generation antipsychotic drugs listed by the BNF (2016)

In addition to the factors listed in Table 6.1, chlorpromazine hydrochloride, haloperidol, pericyazine, perphenazine and trifluoperazine are listed by the BNF (2016) as treatments for "impulsivity/violence". These are not listed as categories of mental illness in the ICD-10 and DSM-5 diagnostic manuals. The same situation exists with benperidol, being recommended as a means of treating antisocial sexual behaviour. Here the BNF notes that this in an "unestablished" form of treatment, therefore one that is to be avoided. The inclusion of pimozide as a means of treating hypochondria seems impossible to justify, given the severe side-effects profile of the drug and credibility of psychological treatment available instead for treating this condition.

Having considered first generation antipsychotic medications, we should next identify second generation antipsychotics and their uses in Table 6.2.

Special consideration must be made when prescribing clozapine. This drug is only deemed suitable for patients experiencing symptoms of schizophrenia that have been unsuccessfully treated by at least two other antipsychotics. This is because of the potential lethality of agranulocytosis, a side-effect resulting in the loss of infection-fighting white blood cells, therefore regular blood tests are required as a prerequisite of clozapine treatment.

Second generation antipsychotics have a reputation for causing fewer side-effects than first generation antipsychotics. In reality this is incorrect, although they may be less severe at lower doses. The common side-effects for all antipsychotic medications are numerous and have significant impact for those using them. Despite being common in practice, prescription of multiple antipsychotics is to be avoided because this intensifies side-effects (Correll et al., 2009).

Original drug name	Alternative names	Recommended as treatment for:
Amisulpride	Solian	Schizophrenia
Aripiprazole	Abilify Abilify Maintena	Schizophrenia Mania Agitation in schizophrenia
Clozapine	Clozaril Denzapine Zaponex	Schizophrenia
Lurasidone hydrochloride	Latuda	Schizophrenia
Olanzapine	Arkolamyl Zalasta Zyprexa	Schizophrenia Mania Bipolar disorder
Paliperidone	Invega Xeplion	Schizophrenia Schizoaffective disorder
Quetiapine	Seroquel Atrolak XL Biquelle XL Ebesque XL Mintreleq XL Psyquet XL Sondate XL Tenprolide XL Zaluron XL	Schizophrenia Bipolar disorder Adjunctive treatment of depression
Risperidone	Risperdal Risperdal Consta	Schizophrenia and other psychosis Mania

Table 6.2: Second generation antipsychotic drugs listed by the BNF (2016)

Perhaps the most striking issues resulting from antipsychotic use are extrapyramidal side-effects. They include tremors and involuntary abnormal movements of the body and face, persistent restlessness, bizarre walk and body posture. Patients may experience tardive dyskinesia, presenting as hard to read facial expressions and peculiar physical presentations. As a result, extrapyramidal side-effects can be socially isolating for people experiencing them. Their impact, once established, is irreversible. Antimuscarinic drugs (typically procyclidine hydrochloride) are routinely prescribed to mask tremors resulting from antipsychotic use. This practice should be avoided because antimuscarinic drugs increase the risk of tardive dyskinesia.

As well as the uniquely debilitating phenomena of extrapyramidal side-effects, many other dangerous side-effects occur through antipsychotic use. Some side-effects impact in multiple ways. For example, reduced **dopamine** levels mean prolactin production is consequentially increased by antipsychotic use. Increased prolactin levels commonly create impotence in men and menstrual disturbances in women, including early onset of menopause. Both genders can experience loss of sex drive, breast enlargement and milk production. Not surprisingly, these side-effects are reported as the most significant in patients choosing to discontinue antipsychotic use. They have a tremendous impact on the self-esteem of the individual and their ability to maintain sexual relationships. Increased prolactin levels also reduce bone density and increase the likelihood of osteoporosis, with concurrent risk of breaking bones from physical injury. Although first generation antipsychotics are renowned for causing these symptoms, they are also particularly associated with amisulpride and risperidone, two second generation drugs.

The experience of sedation may initially be a welcome relief for psychotic patients receiving antipsychotics. For a person with acute symptoms of psychosis, drowsiness may represent an improvement to their current experience of life. However, any longer term assessment of quality of life demonstrates the disastrousness of sedation, present to varying degrees with all antipsychotics. The ability to engage in meaningful conversation, and therefore to develop and maintain relationships is limited. Self-motivation is unlikely to extend sufficiently to enable the person to try new things or seek out the achievement of significant life goals. Despite an increased volume of sleep, the quality experienced is poor, resulting in feelings of perpetual tiredness. Willingness to participate in physical activity of any kind is often limited, with a consequent long-term deterioration of physical wellbeing. The ability to work is likely to be severely affected. Physical activity and achievement of personal ambitions are significant aspects in recovery from severe mental illness (see Chapter 7). **Sedation** therefore presents multiple limiting factors upon long-term recovery and independence from mental health services.

Lack of physical activity resulting from sedation is partially responsible for weight gain common with antipsychotic use. Perhaps more significant are increases in appetite caused by these drugs. Weight gain can be severe, with olanzapine particularly significant in this regard. Weight gain has a detrimental impact on self-esteem, isolating people further who are highly vulnerable in the first place. As well as this psychological aspect, weight gain caused by antipsychotics contributes significantly to the effects of other physical health factors resulting from antipsychotic use.

All antipsychotics are liable to cause hyperglycaemia (excessive glucose in red blood cells) and diabetes. Diabetes is indicated by other symptoms common to antipsychotics, including frequent urination, excessive thirst, blurred vision and fatigue. Hyperglycaemia can cause kidney and nerve damage; diabetes, if untreated, can be fatal. The sedentary lifestyle, and high sugar diet associated with people taking antipsychotics increases the likelihood and impact of these conditions.

A range of dangerous cardiovascular side-effects result from all antipsychotic use. Symptoms include irregular heartbeat (arrhythmias), racing heart (tachycardia), low blood pressure (hypotension) and QT-interval prolongation. Low blood pressure can result in falls, with subsequent injuries, something that is particularly relevant considering the negative effect antipsychotics have on bone density. Low blood pressure can also result in difficulties regulating temperature, hypothermia being potentially fatal. QT-interval prolongation leads to lower heart rate variability, an aspect of cardiac health thought to significantly increase the likelihood of obesity, diabetes and **osteoporosis**, conditions already identified as more prevalent for people being treated with antipsychotics. QT-interval prolongation indicates increased expectancy of arthritis, Alzheimer's disease and cancer (Kemp and Quintana, 2013). QT-interval changes occur with higher than recommended doses of medication, or antipsychotics in depot injection rather than tablet format. Psychological and **cardiovascular** health are positively linked, making these multiple cardiac side-effects counter-indicative to mental health.

All antipsychotics increase their users' photosensitivity, resulting in increased susceptibility to skin cancers. Depletion of vitamin D through avoiding sun exposure should be recognised, as should the social impact of limiting a socially isolated patients' choice of outside activities.

Neuroleptic malignant syndrome is a potentially fatal side-effect possible with any antipsychotic. It is a specific reaction to medication characterised by a combination of sudden and severe changes in mental state, blood pressure readings fluctuating from normal to high, a racing heart, rapid breathing, urinary incontinence and rigidity throughout the muscles of the body. Later stages include fever, but action should be taken before this occurs, as the condition has at this point become severely dangerous.

Caution in prescribing antipsychotics is advised by the BNF (2016) for patients with a range of pre-existing conditions. These include heart or **respiratory** issues, due to the multiple cardiac problems these medications can cause. Pericyazine and prochlorperazine are particularly problematic in this regard, as they have the potential to slow respiratory rates. Patients with Parkinson's disease should avoid antipsychotics due to the potential of worsening tremors. Antipsychotics increase risk of seizures, and therefore should not be prescribed for people who experience epilepsy. There are also links between these medications and jaundice, so they should not be prescribed for patients with a history of this condition. Due to uncertainty concerning their impact, women who are pregnant or are breastfeeding should avoid the use of antipsychotics if at all possible.

Some antipsychotics are provided as an inter-muscular injection (depot) rather than tablet format. Provided it is injected into muscle, the antipsychotic agent is released over a period of weeks into the patient's bloodstream. If depots are administered incorrectly through being injected into fat, they become ineffective. Depot antipsychotics are recommended only to treat schizophrenia or psychosis. Risperidone depot is specified for the treatment of these conditions, and all other depots except fluphenazine are recommended instead for maintenance (prevention of deterioration). The BNF (2016) does not specify whether fluphenazine depot is to be used for maintenance or treatment purposes.

The side-effects of depot medications are largely the same as with tablet forms already discussed, with some additional features. The most significant of these are for fluphenazine depot, including antidiuretic hormone secretion. This results in excess water retention causing lethargy, delirium and confusion. Antidiuretic hormone secretion may therefore be misdiagnosed as symptoms of mental illness. Increasing dosage of fluphenazine depot in an attempt to treat these symptoms makes fluid retention more likely, highlighting the importance of monitoring physical health in psychiatric patients, particularly following prescription changes. Fluphenazine depot may cause systemic lupus erythematosus, a long-term autoimmune condition characterised by joint pain and swelling. This medication may also elevate mood, so is not suitable for patients experiencing mania. Conversely, risperidone depot may cause depression, so is not suitable for patients experiencing psychotic depression, or for many patients with symptoms of low mood as a feature of schizophrenia. Risperidone depot is also known to cause paraesthesia, a condition caused by nerve damage that feels similar to "pins and needles". This is commonly misinterpreted by patients experiencing symptoms of psychosis in a delusional fashion, for example as an insect infestation, so care staff may fail to appreciate it as a side-effect.

Having reviewed the uses and side-effects of antipsychotic medications, we will now consider hypnotic drugs.

Hypnotics

Hypnotic medicines are used in treating insomnia. This consists of severe difficulties achieving or remaining asleep. The main hypnotics identified by the BNF (2016) are listed in Table 6.3.

Original drug name	Alternative names	Recommended as treatment for:
Benzodiazepine hypnotics:		Short-term treatment of insomnia only (specified as two to four weeks).
Flurazepam	Dalmane	
Loprazolam		
Lormetazepam		
Nitrazepam	Mogadon	
Temazepam		
Non-benzodiazepine hypnotics:		Short-term treatment of insomnia
Chloral hydrate		
Clomethiazole	Clomethiazole edisilate	
Melatonin	Circadin	
Zaleplon		Short-term treatment of insomnia for up to two weeks
Zolipidem tartrate	Stilnoct	Short-term treatment of insomnia for up to four weeks
Zopiclone	Zimovane	

Table 6.3: Hypnotic medications listed by the BNF (2016)

As well as the medicines listed in Table 6.3, a few other hypnotic agents are available, but these are rarely used in practice, and so are not discussed here.

In order to be effective, hypnotics must be prescribed for short-term use only. Unfortunately, inappropriate, ongoing prescription of hypnotics is currently widespread in the UK. What should be limited to very short courses of treatment for the most severely distressed individuals has commonly become routine. This is true for patients treated by general practitioners, as well as those in specialist psychiatric services. Rather than being a rare event meeting severest need, prescription of hypnotics remains alarmingly common across the NHS.

All forms of hypnotics are addictive, as tolerance of their effects occurs within days of treatment. This results in limited effectiveness in promoting sleep at original dosages. As a result, withdrawal becomes very difficult. Patients used to relying on hypnotics to achieve sleep initially find attempting rest without them impossible. Withdrawal symptoms may last for weeks, and a properly managed withdrawal process can take up to a year.

Because of the addictiveness of hypnotics, it is critical that caution is observed in their prescription. Prior to prescription, the patient should first undertake serious attempts to establish a healthy sleeping pattern. Other contributory factors, in particular alcohol, need to be ruled out as creating and maintaining insomnia. Ensuring the patient recognises that hypnotics are unlikely to successfully treat chronic insomnia, and will lead to dependency, is critical in enabling an informed decision regarding their use. Most importantly of all, a realistic understanding of the psychological causes of insomnia needs to be recognised by the patient. This is a longer-term solution, and therefore not often favoured by patients seeking short-term relief from symptoms of insomnia.

As well as dependency and withdrawal, benzodiazepine hypnotics also share several other common side-effects. These include ataxia, a temporary abnormality of conditions within the **cerebellum**. This results in an inability to control bodily movements. The range and extent of movements affected varies between individuals, but includes swallowing, walking or talking, and can have minor or severe impact. Because their sedating effects have a tendency to extend into the following day, daytime drowsiness is a common side-effect of all hypnotic benzodiazepines. Patients taking these medications can also become confused and experience partial or full memory loss while under their influence.

The side-effects described for hypnotic benzodiazepines also occur with zolipidem tartrate, as well as a wide range of other common side-effects. This makes it more problematic than other Z-drugs. These include agitation, depression and physical weakness. Double vision, dizziness and falls may take place. The occurrence of paradoxical side-effects mean insomnia can actually be worsened by this drug. Nightmares and sleepwalking have also been reported from zolipidem tartrate use. The patient using this drug may experience diarrhoea, changes to their libido, a rash and tremors.

Whereas zolipidem tartrate has many reported side-effects, zopiclone has very few common problems, principally involving taste disturbances. This positive aspect, and fears concerning the addictiveness of benzodiazepines, make zopiclone a popular choice for prescribers, particularly in primary care. The final Z-drug, zaleplon, also has limited side-effects beyond those shared by all hypnotics. These additions are amnesia, daytime drowsiness, menstrual cramps and paraesthesia.

A number of counter-indications exist for the prescription of hypnotic medications. Since hypnotics cause sedation, they become dangerous for patients with breathing problems, in particular respiratory disease and **acute pulmonary insufficiency**. This is also the case for people with sleep apnoea, as sedation caused by hypnotic medication may dangerously prolong periods the patient spends without breathing. Patients experiencing porphyria, a range of blood disorders, should avoid hypnotics as these drugs may worsen their condition. As hypnotics may cause muscular weakness, people with this kind of pre-existing condition (for example, myasthenia gravis) may find their problems exaggerated when taking these drugs. The addictive nature of hypnotics means they should not be prescribed to people with a history of substance use, or a diagnosis of personality disorder. Patients in this group are often keen to be prescribed hypnotics, so may pressurise prescribers to meet their wishes. Finally, benzodiazepines should not be used in combination with antipsychotic medications, as the latter aggravate benzodiazepine withdrawal symptoms.

Our examination of hypnotic medications concludes with an activity concerning the use of sleeping tablets on a psychiatric unit.

Activity 6.1	*Evidence-based practice*

Imagine that you are a staff nurse working a night shift on an adult inpatient unit. Cyril, a patient with a diagnosis of borderline personality disorder, is currently being treated on an informal basis. He is prescribed a range of medicines including zopiclone 7.5 mg on a PRN basis (medicine provided according to nurse's discretion). You are aware that he has requested this medicine every night since his admission three weeks ago. Other staff members have agreed to his request on a number of occasions. Soon after the start of your shift, Cyril requests his PRN medicine. He tells you that he cannot sleep without this drug, so not giving it to him is against his human rights. How would you respond in this situation?

A suggested answer is provided at the end of this chapter.

The situation described in Activity 6.1 remains a common one, despite the widespread awareness of caution required in providing sleeping tablets. Having examined the uses and health implications of hypnotic medication, we are now able to consider the application and risks involved with anxiolytic medicines. Considerable overlap exists between these two classes of drug.

Anxiolytics

Anxiolytics are a class of drugs recommended principally to treat anxiety. They are mostly benzodiazepines, so are closely related in actions and side-effects to many of the hypnotics previously described, and are presented in Table 6.4.

Original drug name	Alternative names	Recommended as treatment for:
Benzodiazepine anxiolytics		
Alprazolam	Xanax	Short-term treatment of anxiety
Chlordiazepoxide hydrochloride	Librium	
Diazepam	Stesolid	Anxiety, agitation and panic attacks Insomnia Muscular spasm
Lorazepam	Ativan	Short-term treatment of anxiety or insomnia
Oxazepam		
Non-benzodiazepine anxiolytics		
Buspirone hydrochloride		Short-term treatment of anxiety

Table 6.4: Anxiolytic medications listed by the BNF (2016)

As well as the medicines listed in Table 6.4, meprobamate and barbiturates are also forms of anxiolytics, but are not recommended for prescription because the danger of their side-effects outweighs their potential benefit.

Although severity may vary between individuals, side-effect profiles of all benzodiazepine anxiolytics are identical. Although they act over a longer period of time than hypnotics and are therefore less sedating, drowsiness still results from their use. This may lead to confusion and feelings of muscular weakness. Ataxia symptoms are shared with hypnotic benzodiazepines. Paradoxical effects of benzodiazepine anxiolytics may occur, with users becoming more anxious than before receiving treatment. Dependence is common with these drugs.

Buspirone hydrochloride shares drowsiness, muscular weakness and **paradoxical** side-effects with benzodiazepine type anxiolytics. It also causes paraesthesia, but dependency is much less common than is the case with benzodiazepines. Visual disturbances and rash (indicating potential toxicity of treatment) are potential side-effects specific to buspirone hydrochloride.

Counter-indications for anxiolytics are shared with hypnotic benzodiazepines (see p. 120). In addition, benzodiazepine anxiolytics are not recommended for treatment of patients with symptoms of chronic psychosis, anxiety, stress, phobia, complex grief or obsessional states because they have been found to be ineffective in treating these conditions. They should be prescribed at the lowest possible dosage for the shortest time period. This should ideally be between two and four weeks, with strict avoidance of long-term usage. These factors are relevant when undertaking Activity 6.2.

Delbert attends an appointment with his GP requesting medication to help him calm down following several episodes of anxiety. His doctor explains that he is at risk of addiction, therefore prescriptions of this kind are not advisable and treatment through psychological therapy is preferable. Delbert agrees to a referral for CBT and leaves relatively satisfied with this option.

Two weeks later Delbert returns to see his GP. He is significantly distressed, having experienced what he describes as a much more serious panic attack the day before. He also feels that he will be unable to cope with the waiting list for psychological therapies as it is around 16 weeks in his area. His GP reiterates the addictive nature of anxiolytic medicines, but agrees to prescribe Delbert with diazepam on a short-term basis.

Considering all of the factors presenting above, is the doctor correct in his decision?

A suggested answer is presented at the end of this chapter.

Activity 6.2 highlights a regular dilemma in practice between attempts to prevent suffering, and risks in taking anxiolytic medicines. Having considered the impact of anxiolytic drugs, we may now review health risks of drugs used for the treatment of mania and hypomania.

Drugs used for the treatment of mania and hypomania

In practice, these drugs are often termed "mood stabilisers". They are listed in Table 6.5.

Original drug name	Alternative names	Recommended as treatment for:
Asenapine	Sycrest	Manic symptoms
Carbamazepine		
Lithium carbonate	Camcolit Liskonum Priadel	Manic symptoms Depression Self-mutilation Aggression
Lithium citrate	Li-Liquid Priadel liquid	
Valproic acid	Convulex Depakote	Manic symptoms

Table 6.5: Medications listed by the BNF (2016) for treatment of mania and hypomania

In addition to the factors listed in Table 6.5, carbamazepine is specified for situations where other treatments have failed. The side-effect profiles of these drugs vary considerably, except for lithium carbonate and lithium citrate, which are identical. For ease of description, they will henceforth be described here as "lithium". Asenapine and valproic acid provide fewer issues than other drugs in this class, but their side-effects remain extremely dangerous.

Carbamazepine can precipitate several debilitating blood conditions. Aplastic anaemia causes deficiency of red and white blood cells and platelets, so negatively impacts a range of bodily systems. Carbamazepine may also damage bone marrow and hematopoietic stem cells. This destruction of red blood cells may create fatigue, heart arrhythmias, enlarged heart and heart failure. White blood cells may increase in number (eosinophilia) due to an allergy to carbamazepine, or they may decrease in numbers, causing vulnerability to infection. This drug may result in thrombocytopenia (low blood platelet count), reducing the ability for blood to clot following injury. Thrombocytopenia may also occur for patients taking valproic acid.

Lithium use may increase white blood cells (leucocytosis), due to the poisonous nature of the drug. This causes multiple muscular-skeletal issues. These include arthralgia (painful joints) and myalgia (painful muscles), muscular weakness and hyperparathyroidism (and excess calcium in the blood that weakens bones). Lithium and carbamazepine cause oedema, indicating a potentially fatal allergy to these medicines. Asenapine may cause **paraesthesia**, indicating potential nerve damage, and rhabdomyolysis (extensive muscle damage throughout the body).

Lithium may create diabetic symptoms in the patient. They may experience great thirst (polydipsia), pass excessive amounts of urine (polyuria) and develop excessive levels of bloodstream glucose (hyperglycaemia). Because carbamazepine creates the diabetic symptom of dry mouth, patients using it should also be monitored for diabetes.

Asenapine has the potential to create a number of oral health issues. These include swollen or painful tongue (glossodynia), difficulty swallowing (dysphagia), taste disturbances and oral hypoaesthesia (reduced sense of touch in the mouth). Carbamazepine can also create skin conditions (dermatitis) and intensely itchy red welts and swelling of the skin (urticaria), caused by an allergic reaction. Valproic acid use can lead to hair loss. Oral, skin and hair condition are important indicators of overall physical wellbeing. The side-effects described indicate the toxic impact of medications throughout the systems of the body.

Gastrointestinal disturbances are common to all mania and hypomania treatments except for asenapine. Lithium and valproic acid cause diarrhoea and other less specific gastro-intestinal issues. Lithium and carbamazepine may cause vomiting, with nausea reported from carbamazepine and valproic acid. Dehydration caused by diarrhoea or sickness may be particularly dangerous in combination with other blood chemistry issues occurring as side-effects of these medicines.

Depending on the patient, lithium use can result in either loss of appetite or weight gain. The latter symptom is also a potential of valproic acid. Rapid weight changes indicate poor mental health and are symptoms of depression.

Lithium can create speech difficulties (shared with asenapine) and visual disturbances and kidney impairment through toxic overload. Carbamazepine is known to cause headaches. Because of the toxicity of these compounds, any of these symptoms potentially indicate highly dangerous trauma to the brain.

The paradoxical side-effect of anxiety can be caused by asenapine. Hyperthyroidism can result from lithium use, causing weight loss, a rapid or irregular heartbeat and sweating. Lithium can create nervousness or irritability which are symptoms used to diagnose mania. These side-effects can be misinterpreted as psychological in cause, leading to increasing dosages when they should be reduced, with further harm to the patient.

Carbamazepine and lithium may result in a number of issues related to movement, which may be misinterpreted as symptoms of mental disorder. Both medicines can create ataxia, the loss of control of bodily movements. Lithium can create tremors, and carbamazepine can create dizziness, drowsiness and fatigue.

The use of lithium has specific cautions. It is hazardous in combination with haloperidol and flupentixol. Concurrent use of diuretics and lithium is hazardous, as sodium depletion worsens damage done through lithium overdose. Lithium is only recommended in treating acute mania if the patient has severe symptoms and has responded to lithium before. Long-term use may result in thyroid disorders and cognitive impairment. To avoid overdose, the concentration of lithium in the patient's blood needs regular monitoring, presenting a risk factor for patients who are unwilling or unable to maintain regular contact with mental health services.

Having explored the uses and potential side-effects of drugs prescribed for the treatment of mania and hypomania, Activity 6.3 considers their use in practice.

Activity 6.3 — *Evidence-based practice*

Cecilia is a woman with a diagnosis of bipolar disorder who has been prescribed carbamazepine for almost ten years. Her community mental health team report that she has moved from a period of high energy, to one of low mood, as she has become uncharacteristically **lethargic**.

In order to rule out non-psychological causes of Cecilia's change in mental wellbeing, a review of her care is undertaken by her treatment team. Because of her presentation, which side-effects require further investigation?

A suggested answer is presented at the end of this chapter.

The symptoms experienced by Cecilia demonstrate why prescribing psychotropic medicine requires consideration of multiple factors, often beyond the obvious.

Our exploration of medicines used for the treatment of psychological symptoms concludes with a review of antidepressant medication, perhaps the commonest form of prescription for mental health issues.

Antidepressant medication

A large proportion of medicines prescribed in both primary care and specialist mental health practice comprise of antidepressants. These medicines belong to one of four groups. These are termed tricyclic and related antidepressants, monoamine-oxidase inhibitors (MAOIs) and reversible MAOIs, selective serotonin re-uptake inhibitors (SSRIs), and other antidepressant drugs. Each of these four groups will now be considered in turn.

Tricyclic and tricyclic related antidepressants

Tricyclic and tricyclic related medicines (known henceforth as tricyclics) are the oldest form of antidepressants. They are listed in Table 6.6.

Caution is advised when prescribing tricyclic medications for patients with cardiovascular issues, hyperthyroidism, epilepsy, diabetes, phaeochromocytoma (tumour of the adrenal glands) and antimuscarinic activity (primarily because of issues regarding dilation of the pupils).

Original drug name	Alternative names	Recommended as treatment for:
Amitriptyline hydrochloride	Triptafen	Depression
Clomipramine hydrochloride		Depression Phobic and obsessional states
Dosulepin hydrochloride	Dothiepin hydrochloride Prothiaden	Depression
Doxepin		
Imipramine hydrochloride	Imipramine	
Lofepramine	Lofepramine hydrochloride Lomont	
Mianserin hydrochloride	Mianserin	
Nortriptyline	Nortriptyline hydrochloride	
Trazodone hydrochloride	Molipaxin	
Trimipramine	Trimipramine maleate	

Table 6.6: Tricyclic and tricyclic related antidepressants listed by the BNF (2016)

This is because tricyclic medications can directly worsen these conditions through multiple side-effects resulting from their use.

A major drawback to the use of tricyclics is their high risk of fatality in overdose, especially with dosulepin hydrochloride and amitriptyline hydrochloride. Tricyclics are therefore not recommended for patients at high risk of suicide, or with a history of bipolar disorder or other psychosis. This factor limits their prescription in clinical practice.

The side-effects of tricyclic medication are considerable. Those common to all medicines in this class include breast enlargement (gynaecomastia) and production of milk (gallactorrhoea) within both genders, **convulsions**, dry mouth (suggesting diabetes), blurred vision (also a symptom of high blood sugar) and urinary retention. A range of further side-effects exist for each individual medicine.

Issues related to the circulatory system are created by tricyclic antidepressants. These include hypertension (increased blood pressure) from taking clomipramine hydrochloride and nortriptyline. Hypertension may also be indicated by headaches and heart palpitations (rapid, strong or irregular heartbeat) from imipramine hydrochloride use. Priapism (an unwanted, painful erection that may cause erectile dysfunction) can occur with any tricyclic, but in particular trazodone hydrochloride. As priapism is caused by narrowing of the arteries, it indicates further issues with the person's cardiovascular system. This drug can also cause dyspnoea (difficulty breathing), making it harder to supply oxygen throughout the body. Blood dyscrasias, an imbalance between plasma, white and red blood cells, can be a side-effect of mianserin hydrochloride. Any tricyclic may cause dizziness, **arrhythmia**, **heartblock**, tachycardia and ECG changes.

Gastro-intestinal problems caused by clomipramine hydrochloride, doxepin and nortriptyline include abdominal pain and diarrhoea. Other tricyclics may cause constipation. Trazodone hydrochloride may cause indigestion (dyspepsia).

Tricyclics can cause a range of muscular-skeletal problems. Mianserin hydrochloride may cause arthralgia (joint pain) and arthritis (this also occurs with mianserin hydrochloride). Muscular weakness, hypertonia (stiffness, indicating nerve damage) and myoclonus (spasmodic contraction of muscles) can result from taking clomipramine hydrochloride, with myalgia (muscular pain) possible from trazodone hydrochloride use.

Lofepramine, mianserin hydrochloride and trazodone hydrochloride may cause liver dysfunction. This may be indicated through **jaundice** or **hypersalivation**. Flushing skin is often wrongly overlooked as a harmless side-effect of clomipramine hydrochloride, doxepin, imipramine hydrochloride and nortriptyline, but in fact may indicate palpations of the liver.

Doxepin and nortriptyline may cause stomatitis (an inflamed mouth). This not only affects the ability to eat, talk and sleep, but may also represent a serious allergy to treatment. These tricyclic drugs, along with lofepramine and mianserin hydrochloride, can cause oedema (swelling of body tissues, indicating potentially fatal allergies from treatment).

Mydriasis (dilation of the pupil) caused by clomipramine hydrochloride or nortriptyline can signify raised intraocular pressure in the eye. This is one of the main risk factors for glaucoma. Raised intraocular pressure may occur directly as a result of taking amitriptyline hydrochloride or dosulepin hydrochloride. All tricyclics can lead to changes in blood sugar, increased appetite and weight gain, making diabetes more likely in the user. Paradoxically, these drugs can instead result in weight loss or anorexia (loss of appetite) for other patients.

A number of side-effects caused by these drugs can be mistaken for psychiatric symptoms, possibly resulting in inappropriate prescription of other medicines. Clomipramine hydrochloride may cause aggression, memory impairment, restlessness or fatigue (this last issue also occurs with imipramine hydrochloride). All tricyclics can cause psychiatric symptoms in the form of anxiety, hallucinations, delusions, mania or hypomania. Sedation, sleep disturbances, drowsiness, irritability and confusion may also occur, making tricyclic antidepressants problematic for prescribers. Awareness that these drugs can cause sexual dysfunction is important for healthcare professionals because this is a primary cause of patients discontinuing their use.

Monoamine-oxidase inhibitors (MAOIs) and reversible MAOIs

Monoamine-oxidase inhibitors were developed as an alternative to tricyclic antidepressants, and were initially popular with prescribers due to being less dangerous in overdose. Combination of tricyclic and MAOI use is, however, potentially fatal. MAOIs may increase blood pressure when taken in conjunction with alcohol, cough remedies and decongestants, and many food groups containing yeast, such as cheese, Bovril, Oxo and Marmite. Fish and meat products that are "going off" may also cause these reactions. MAOIs are listed in Table 6.7.

MAOIs cause cardiovascular side-effects. **Postural hypotension** is caused by phenelzine, isocarboxazid and tranylcypromine. This may explain the occurrence of dizziness from all MAOIs. Tranylcypromine has the potential to cause hypertensive crisis, a severe increase in blood pressure that damages blood vessels and causes stroke. This drug may also cause **blood dyscrasias**.

Moclobemide creates side-effects which may be misinterpreted as psychiatric symptoms. These include agitation, sleep disturbances and confusion. Tranylcypromine can create **insomnia**. Any of these side-effects can result in prescription of additional medication in an attempt to counteract these symptoms.

Original drug name	Alternative names	Recommended as treatment for:
Isocarboxazid		Depression
Moclobemide	Manerix	Depression Social anxiety disorder
Phenelzine	Nardil	Depression
Tranylcypromine		

Table 6.7: MAOI and reversible MAOI antidepressants listed by the BNF (2016)

Moclobemide creates a number of indicators of toxicity, including headaches, paraesthesia, skin reactions, gastro-intestinal disorders and **oedema**. Phenelzine and isocarboxazid are MAOIs that more frequently cause liver damage, with tranylcypromine doing so less often. Moclobemide use may lead to side-effects of dry mouth and visual disturbances that are synonymous with diabetes.

Selective serotonin re-uptake inhibitors (SSRIs)

Case study: Eleanor

Eleanor is prescribed sertraline following a period of anxiety and low mood. Rather than feeling better, she feels even worse after taking this medicine. Her poor state of mind means that she does not want to make a fuss, so despite feeling physically unwell she persists with treatment. On review, her GP diagnoses postural hypotension and tachycardia as side-effects of sertraline use.

The side-effects experienced by Eleanor are relatively common. Her situation is an example of some of the limiting factors of SSRIs as treatment for depression. The side-effects apparent from this most widely prescribed class of antidepressants are considerable.

SSRIs are the latest development in antidepressant medication, and are normally the first choice of treatment for prescribing doctors. Medications in this group are listed in Table 6.8.

Caution is advised in prescribing SSRIs for patients who are epileptic or receiving electro convulsive therapy, have heart conditions, diabetes, glaucoma, gastro-intestinal or bleeding issues. These medications are not suitable for patients with a history of mania because of the further elevation of mood that may result from SSRI use.

SSRIs share a number of common side-effects. These include sedation, cardiovascular issues, gastro-intestinal problems (such as indigestion, constipation or diarrhoea, nausea and vomiting), disturbances of appetite and bodyweight, muscular and joint pains, and anaphylaxis (a potentially fatal reaction due to toxicity of the medicines taken).

Multiple cardiovascular side-effects result from SSRI use. Heart palpitations are reported for all drugs except for escitalopram and paroxetine. Citalopram can cause bradycardia (an abnormally slow heart), hypokalaemia (low blood potassium levels, affecting heart function), **QT interval prolongation** and postural hypotension (this also occurs with sertraline use). Despite its potential to cause bradycardia, citalopram can also cause tachycardia (an abnormally fast resting heart rate). Tachycardia may also occur from fluvoxamine maleate or sertraline use. Fluvoxamine maleate may cause chills, possibly due to vasodilation (a widening of blood vessels that can cause hypothermia), or a narrowing of the arteries indicated by priapism. Hypercholesterolaemia (high fat levels in the blood) and hypertension may result from paroxetine or sertraline use.

A range of oral health issues can result from SSRI medications. Fluoxetine can cause dysphagia (difficulty swallowing), pharyngitis (sore throat) and taste disturbances. This last symptom is also

Original drug name	Alternative names	Recommended as treatment for:
Citalopram	Cipramil	Depression Panic disorder
Escitalopram	Cipralex	Depression Panic disorder Social anxiety disorder
Fluoxetine	Olena Oxactin Prozac Prozep	Depression Bulimia nervosa Obsessive-compulsive disorder
Fluvoxamine maleate	Favein	Depression Obsessive-compulsive disorder
Paroxetine	Seroxat	Depression Panic disorder Social anxiety disorder Post-traumatic stress disorder Generalised anxiety disorder Obsessive-compulsive disorder
Sertraline	Lustral	Depression Panic disorder Social anxiety disorder Post-traumatic stress disorder Obsessive-compulsive disorder

Table 6.8: SSRI antidepressants listed by the BNF (2016)

caused by citalopram, as well as excessive saliva and a sore mouth. Escitalopram use can result in inflamed sinuses.

Fluoxetine can result in dyspnoea (difficulty breathing) or inflamed lungs, and sertraline can create bronchospasm (mild to severe breathing difficulties).

Liver issues may occur through taking SSRIs. Hepatitis (inflammation of the liver) can result from citalopram, fluoxetine and sertraline use. Sertraline may also cause jaundice or liver failure. Flushing, and pruritus, an urge to scratch, may indicate liver dysfunction from fluoxetine use.

Migraine, coughing and rhinitis (inflamed mucous membranes of the nose) resulting from citalopram use have multiple causes, but can indicate allergic reactions. Toxicity may be a possible cause of pyrexia (raised body temperature or fever) from escitalopram use, and diarrhoea from fluoxetine. Neuroleptic malignant syndrome (presenting as fever, muscular rigidity, altered mental state, and postural or seated hypotension) resulting from an allergic reaction to fluoxetine, can be fatal. Further evidence of fluoxetine's toxicity is presented through the occurrence of alopecia (hair loss) and potentially fatal toxic epidermal necrosis (**lesions** of the skin, gastro-intestinal **haemorrhage**, respiratory failure, **ocular** abnormalities and **genitourinary** complications). Issues with the user's central nervous system may be linked to **toxicity**, for example paraesthesia caused by citalopram, escitalopram or sertraline use.

Citalopram may cause micturition disorders (blood in the urine), potentially due to haemorrhage of blood vessels. This issue is also possible with fluoxetine. Leucopenia (decreased white blood cells, essential for autoimmunity) can be a side-effect of sertraline.

Symptoms indicating poor general health through SSRI use include fatigue (caused by escitalopram) and **tinnitus** (signifying a problem with circulation) resulting from citalopram or sertraline use. Malaise, an experience of bodily weakness, can result from citalopram, fluoxetine or fluvoxamine maleate use.

A variety of symptoms relating to diabetes may occur through SSRI use. Citalopram can create mydriasis (dilated pupils, possibly indicating raised intraocular pressure) or polyuria (frequent urination, a common indicator of diabetes). This symptom is shared with fluoxetine, which also leads to blood sugar changes. Hypoglycaemia can result from sertraline use; this constitutes abnormally low blood glucose levels causing headaches, confusion, irrational behaviour, unconsciousness, **seizure** or coma.

Diagnosable psychiatric symptoms may occur through SSRI use. Sleep disturbances, confusion and impaired concentration may result from citalopram and fluoxetine use, as well as yawning indicating drowsiness (this also occurs with escitalopram and paroxetine). Citalopram may cause aggression, amnesia and paradoxical anxiety. These symptoms are shared with sertraline, which may also result in hypothyroidism. Escitalopram can cause restlessness. Resulting nervousness and irritability may be misinterpreted as symptoms of mania, as can **euphoria** created by citalopram or fluoxetine use. Other factors that may be damaging to the self-esteem of the user include **hyperprolactinaemia** and menstrual irregularities (heavy, irregular or absent menstrual periods) through sertraline use.

Other antidepressant drugs

A number of other medications that do not belong in the antidepressant groups already covered are listed in Table 6.9.

Cautions for prescription of this class of drugs are individualised, complex and therefore beyond the scope of this book. Readers should refer to the BNF (2016) for more information. Side-effects for these drugs vary considerably between medicines. Because flupentixol is used primarily as an antipsychotic, it has been discussed previously (see p. 114).

Medications within this group include considerable cardiovascular side-effects. Reboxetine and mirtazapine cause **hypotension**, which may also be the cause of dizziness symptoms from

Original drug name	Alternative names	Recommended as treatment for:
Agomelatine	Valdoxan	Depression
Duloxetine	Cymbalta Duciltia Yentreve	Depression Generalised anxiety disorder
Flupentixol	Fluanxol Depixol	See Table 6.1, p. 114
Mirtazapine	Zispin SolTab	Depression
Reboxetine	Edronax	Depression
Tryptophan	L-tryptophan Optimax	Depression
Venlafaxine	Alventa XL Amphero XL Depefex XL Efexor XL Politid XL Rodomel XL Sunveniz XL Tonpular XL Venaxx XL Venlablue XL Venladex XL Venlalic XL Venlaneo XL Vensir XL Vexarin XL ViePax XL	Depression Generalised anxiety disorder Social anxiety disorder

Table 6.9: Other antidepressant drugs listed by the BNF (2016)

agomelatine and venlafaxine use. Heart palpitations may result from reboxetine and venlafaxine use, with the former also causing tachycardia. Flupentixol may cause Torsade de pointes, a particularly dangerous form of tachycardia. This medication may also create dyspnoea (breathing difficulties). Serum transaminases (an enzyme present through agomelatine use) indicate heart damage. Venlafaxine can cause increases in blood cholesterol, with consequent impact on cardiovascular disease. Other conditions relating to the venous system include **vasodilation** from reboxetine and venlafaxine use.

Mirtazapine may lead to arthralgia (joint pain) and myalgia (muscular pain). Flupentixol also creates this latter issue. Venlafaxine can create hypertonia (increased muscle tone and inability to stretch caused by nerve damage). This may explain back pain associated with agomelatine use. A range of further issues relating to the central nervous system are also possible from these medicines. Impotence and urinary retention from reboxetine use may be due to nerve damage. This drug, along with agomelatine, causes sweating that may result from an overactive sympathetic nervous system. Venlafaxine may cause tremor and disturbances of the senses (sight, sound, smell, taste, temperature, pain and body movements). Tremor may also occur with mirtazapine use.

Flupentixol may cause sudden death and has higher withdrawal risks than other antidepressants. Visual disturbances resulting from reboxetine and venlafaxine, or mydriasis (fixed dilated pupils) from venlafaxine use may indicate serotinin syndrome, a potentially fatal condition.

Symptoms of toxicity include confusion caused by mirtazapine and venlafaxine, vomiting from agomelatine and venlafaxine, and nausea resulting from agomelatine, reboxetine and venlafaxine use. Agomelatine may cause abdominal pain, diarrhoea or constipation. This last symptom also occurs with reboxetine and venlafaxine use.

Diabetic symptoms resulting from the consumption of this class of medicines include hyperglycaemia (high blood sugar levels) resulting from flupentixol use. Dry mouth experienced through mirtazapine, reboxetine and venlafaxine use may indicate diabetes. Increased appetite occurring with mirtazapine is also a strong indicator of diabetes.

Side-effects that may be misinterpreted as psychological symptoms are particularly prevalent in this group of medicines. Drowsiness is common with agomelatine, mirtazapine and venlafaxine. Insomnia can be a side-effect of reboxetine, mirtazapine and venlafaxine. The latter two medicines may also cause nightmares and anxiety. Reboxetine and venlafaxine may cause significant loss of appetite. Agitation may result from agomelatine use. The effects of withdrawal are more significant for venlafaxine than for other antidepressants.

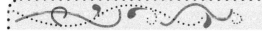

Chapter summary

Our review of psychiatric medicines has highlighted the remarkably toxic nature of these substances. Although side-effects vary, they typically represent chronic debilitation of a range of physiological systems. They may also involve acute toxicity, with potentially fatal consequences. Although every practitioner working in mental health services has some awareness of the side-effects of psychiatric medication, the significance of their toxicity is rarely appreciated. There are very few examples in practice of patients being supported through mental crises without prescription of the medicines described in this chapter. This situation is ethically indefensible because very few practitioners are suitably aware of side-effect profiles to accurately inform their patients of the health risks they are taking from this treatment. It is imperative for the future credibility of mental health services for this situation to change. Full patient involvement in decision-making is necessary concerning psychiatric medications.

Activities: brief outline answers

Activity 6.1 Evidence-based practice (page 121)

It appears that Cyril is developing a dependence on zopiclone in order to sleep. The nature of Cyril's mental health issues suggests that this is particularly likely to be the case. We have a duty of care in this situation to empower him to take appropriate responsibility for his own health. It is important to ensure that Cyril adopts a more realistic and healthy approach to sleep, rather than relying on artificial means of doing so. By denying this medication, a health promotional message is sent which must be supported through development of an evidence-based care plan by Cyril and the multi-disciplinary team. Cyril is a reminder for the care team regarding the likelihood of patients becoming unnecessarily reliant on hypnotic medication.

Activity 6.2 Evidence-based practice (page 123)

Delbert certainly seems to be in considerable need of assistance with anxiety issues that are having a significant impact on the quality of his life. His doctor is seeking to alleviate his suffering, but in fact is not acting in his best interests. Anxiolytic medication must be used in the extremely short term only. Prescribing it as a means of supporting him while he waits to begin psychotherapy is unwise, as this time period far exceeds recommendations for anxiolytic use. Delbert's GP has an important role in ensuring that he does not also become dependent on anxiolytic treatment. A useful option prior to commencing CBT would be for his doctor to refer Delbert to a support group for anxiety, if available in his local area.

Activity 6.3 Evidence-based practice (page 125)

Because Cecilia is being treated with carbamazepine, her care plan should indicate that this medicine may cause bone marrow and hematopoietic stem cells damage. If this is the case, she will be feeling fatigue due to loss of red blood cells. If heart arrhythmias are also present after testing, the cause of fatigue as a side-effect of carbamazepine becomes more likely. Fatigue is a useful warning in these circumstances because it may signal the development of other potentially fatal heart conditions.

Further reading

The Cochrane Library is a free of charge database of health research undertaken using the strictest methodological criteria. They include the most thoroughly researched appraisals of the effectiveness of psychiatric medications. Some examples relevant to medicines used in mental health practice include:

Hamann J, Kissling W, Leucht S and Rummel-Kluge C (2003) *New generation antipsychotics for first episode schizophrenia.* Cochrane Database of Systematic Reviews 2003, Issue 4.

Purgato M, Papola D, Gastaldon C, Trespidi C, Magni LR, Rizzo C, Furukawa TA, Watanabe N, Cipriani A and Barbui C (2014) *Paroxetine versus other anti-depressive agents for depression.* Cochrane Database of Systematic Reviews April 3(4).

Appendix A **of the BNF** (2016) is invaluable for consultation in order to appreciate if any of the medicines prescribed to patients are known to interact unfavourably with each other. This resource has developed over time, based on reports of adverse drug interactions provided by health practitioners using the Yellow Card Scheme described in the BNF (2016).

NICE guidelines indicate best practice concerning the use of psychiatric medications for a range of common mental health issues. For example, see:

National Institute for Health and Care Excellence (2014) *Clinical Guidelines [CG178] Psychosis and Schizophrenia* (updated March 2014).

National Institute for Clinical Excellence (2009) *Clinical Guidelines [CG90] Depression in Adults: Recognition and Management* (updated April 2016).

Chapter 7
Recovery from mental health problems

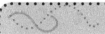 NMC Standards for Pre-registration Nursing Education

This chapter will address the following competencies:

Domain 1: Professional values

4. All nurses must work in partnership with service users, carers, groups, communities and organisations. They must manage risk, and promote health and wellbeing while aiming to empower choices that promote self-care and safety.

4.1 Mental health nurses must work with people in a way that values, respects and explores the meaning of their individual lived experiences of mental health problems, to provide person-centred and recovery-focused practice.

Domain 2: Communication and interpersonal skills

5.1 Mental health nurses must use their personal qualities, experiences and interpersonal skills to develop and maintain therapeutic, recovery-focused relationships with people and therapeutic groups. They must be aware of their own mental health, and know when to share aspects of their own life to inspire hope while maintaining professional boundaries.

6.1 Mental health nurses must foster helpful and enabling relationships with families, carers and other people important to the person experiencing mental health problems. They must use communication skills that enable psychosocial education, problem-solving and other interventions to help people cope and to safeguard those who are vulnerable.

Domain 3: Nursing practice and decision-making

9.1 Mental health nurses must use recovery-focused approaches to care in situations that are potentially challenging, such as times of acute distress; when compulsory measures are used; and in forensic mental health settings. They must seek to maximise service user involvement and therapeutic engagement, using interventions that balance the need for safety with positive risk-taking.

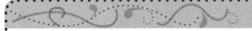

NMC Essential Skills Clusters

This chapter will address the following ESC:

Cluster: Care, compassion and communication

2.4   Actively supports people in their own care and self-care.

2.8   Is sensitive and empowers people to meet their own needs and make choices and considers with the person and their carer(s) their capability to care.

2.14 Actively helps people to identify and use their strengths to achieve their goals and aspirations.

Chapter aims

By the end of the chapter you will be able to:

* understand the philosophy of care supporting recovery-based rehabilitation, and explain it to patients, families and colleagues;
* recognise treatment processes used in recovery-based services;
* appreciate fundamental disputes between traditional psychiatry and recovery-focused practice, despite claims of compatibility made in mental health service policies;
* apply recovery principles to your work with service users.

Introduction

Case study: Michelle

Darren is a newly qualified staff nurse working in an inpatient psychiatric ward. One of the longer-term patients, Michelle, is being treated for schizophrenia. Issues finding her a suitably supportive community placement have made her stay in hospital longer than anticipated. As a consequence, Michelle has lost confidence concerning tasks of daily living, such as cooking, cleaning and shopping. In their work together, Darren and Michelle recognise her need to regain independence through practising tasks of daily living. Together they develop a plan of daily activity that begins with joint trips to the nearby corner shop, and develops into Michelle visiting the local town for a longer shopping trip. This plan provides considerable development for Michelle, as she hasn't left the hospital grounds alone since her admission, and requires her to have faith in Darren's support. Darren records in the team diary their daily trips during the following week.

> *When he arrives on his next shift, Darren finds his notes crossed out. He asks if anyone knows why this is the case and Gareth, one of the senior staff nurses on duty, tells him "I cancelled it because I can't spare you away from the ward." Darren disputes this, as the unit is settled and well-staffed. He is told that this decision is necessary in case anything happens and "going to the shop with patients is not important and they can go themselves". Darren is frustrated by this as he feels that Michelle's efforts to undertake positive risk-taking have been undermined through his colleagues' lack of appreciation of the recovery process. Michelle feels unable to visit the shop alone and is relieved by Gareth's decision because she would rather continue to avoid leaving the hospital grounds.*

Michelle's situation illustrates differences between traditional psychiatry and recovery-focused mental health work. Darren recognises the value in helping patients to push themselves towards recovery through positive risk-taking, whereas Gareth presents an old-fashioned approach to care where patients are required to passively accept treatment based on psychiatric medication. Despite recovery being recognised as a valuable approach by mental health experts, it is underused in many practice areas.

Recovery is a concept which has featured extensively in mental health literature since the 1990s. It is a perennial focus of mental health policy, and in strategic design of local practice areas. This is surprising because there is no consensus of what recovery is, what it aims for, or how it is brought about. The individualised nature of recovery as a process of self-determination makes it distinct for each individual undertaking it. Rather than attempting to pin down a universal definition of recovery, this chapter looks at the philosophy of recovery and methods of delivery in practice, so that practitioners can facilitate recovery wherever possible. Claims that traditional mental health systems are recovery-focused are disputed. Differing approaches to recovery are considered, including recovery as an absence of symptoms and as a process of personal development. Factors necessary in enabling recovery and operationalising recovery are discussed. Recovery is influenced by many aspects of care, including the housing and criminal justice systems, friends and family influences, and physical health. The impact of therapy, social networks, personal productivity, identity, spirituality and healthy lifestyle are all relevant to enabling recovery. Recovery from symptoms of mental ill health and recovery from addiction are considered as interconnected processes in this chapter, as the overlap between mental distress and addiction is significant.

Psychiatric versus recovery perspectives

Psychiatry is a branch of medicine focusing on treatment of mental disorders. It attempts to redress proposed biochemical abnormalities within the brains of its patients through prescribing a range of drugs that impact on the central nervous system. It is a hierarchical approach to treatment that allows psychiatrists to detain patients, when necessary, using the Mental Health Act (1983). Psychiatry and recovery are approaches that are fundamentally opposed to each other. This is because "recovery is about changing the person's life not about changing their **biochemistry**", whereas psychiatry seeks chemical rebalance in the brains of the patient (Montellano, 2015, p. 190). Recovery therefore represents a paradigm shift from traditional mental health provision. This is because poor patient outcomes lead a medically dominated psychiatric system to expect long-term disability following the development of severe mental health issues (Tiderington, 2015). This misconception is based on clinical experiences based on medications that at best stabilise patients' conditions rather than cure their symptoms. Because most services work with people when they are acutely unwell, this lowers clinical expectations in mental health staff by creating the "clinicians' illusion" that change is not possible (Cohen and Cohen, 1984, in Leith, 2014). Low expectations in psychiatry contradict the hope, sense of purpose and ability to change that are central to the recovery ethos. Responsibility is placed on the recovering person to own their recovery process by living the changes they need to become healthy. In contrast, the psychiatric system takes responsibility for change from patients, through the assumption that symptoms of mental disorder limit their ability to make their own decisions. The recovery approach suggests significant change is possible for anybody, whereas psychiatric prognosis is extremely poor. In contrast, results of recovery-focused mental healthcare are commonly successful (Leith, 2014). Although the picture is mixed, many current mental health services do not prioritise the recovery approach.

The primary and dominant aim of modern psychiatric practice is the prevention of suicide. A secondary aim is to treat service users in a manner that makes them well, with an acceptance that this is rarely possible because of the ineffectiveness of the medical approach. The further reading section in Chapter 6 (p. 134) lists several Cochrane reviews demonstrating the lack of robust evidence supporting medicines in psychiatry. Recovery from a psychiatric perspective may involve better management of symptoms specified by ICD-10 or DSM-V manuals. It could also result in a decrease of suicidal ideas which had caused concern for the patient, their family, or health professionals; or it could mean the physical survival of a person following a suicide attempt (Heller, 2015; Myers et al., 2016). These are reactive aims based on negative events, failing to nurture the patient's strengths. In contrast, recovery services highlight development of personal assets as critical in creating lasting change. The possibility of self-harm and suicide make psychiatry a risk-averse approach, contrasting with the positive risk-taking which forms the basis of the recovery concept.

Psychiatric practice defines patients according to broad categories of illness determined by their symptoms. People are grouped according to abnormal emotional and psychological characteristics, such as depressed, psychotic or personality disordered types. Psychiatric medication is inflexible in its application, being available in a limited range of doses, with some medicines prescribed across a range of conditions. Recovery entirely opposes this production line approach to treatment, instead emphasising individual recovery needs and experiences. Recovery is a complex non-linear process that contrasts with the simplistic assumption in psychiatry that the patient is either "ill" or "well". Many patients report experiences of this type to be incredibly debilitating (Tiderington, 2015). The individuality of a recovery experience allows only the individual themselves to accurately judge if they are functioning adequately. This viewpoint may be challenging for mental health staff used to making decisions on behalf of their patients.

The recovery experience varies greatly between individuals, with self-directed change rather than professional input central to effective progress (Anthony, 1993). Belief in the self as primary agent of change contrasts with most mental health practice, where many decisions are made by the health professionals on their patients' behalf. This way of working is based on a belief that individuals with mental health issues overwhelmingly lack the capacity to make decisions for their own benefit, and that mental health staff are instead equipped to make decisions for them. This approach is unnecessarily risk-averse, and therefore counterproductive in supporting recovery. Psychiatric practice is fundamentally opposed to Davidson and Roe's model of recovery, where autonomy in identifying personally determined goals is central to mental wellbeing following experiences of mental ill health (Davidson and Roe, 2007, in Myers et al., 2016).

Psychiatry seeks to stabilise its patients through medication and enforced hospitalisation. In contrast, recovery-informed services seek to improve mental health through facilitating individually determined change, regardless of current symptoms. The possibility of relapse is not a reason to delay undertaking recovery-centred care. The philosophy of personal independence central to recovery means that it cannot thrive in the risk-averse psychiatric system that predominates in twenty-first-century mental healthcare. Activity 7.1 asks you to consider the process and impact of moving to a recovery-focused system of mental health provision.

Activity 7.1   *Decision-making*

Issues with making recovery-focused care a reality in clinical practice

From what we have discussed so far, it is clear that there are major clashes between standard psychiatric treatment and recovery-focused approaches. Consider what you could do to enable transformation of your practice area to adopt a recovery focus. What implications would this have for your patients and colleagues? Review your answer at the end of the chapter to see how your views have changed.

Because of the individual nature of your practice circumstances, an outline answer is not provided at the end of this chapter.

This activity illustrates that many of the changes necessary to enable recovery involve risk-taking. With this in mind, it is appropriate to now consider positive risk-taking as a central component of recovery.

Positive risk-taking as a recovery factor

The differences between standard psychiatry and recovery-focused practice are a result of varying views on what is achievable in mental healthcare. Central in this regard is risk. During a period of mental disruption, a person may undertake behaviour that is highly risky for their health (for example, drug taking, being overly trusting of others financially or sexually, self-harming). Alternatively, they may become highly risk-avoidant, particularly concerning social experiences (such as avoiding friends or family, refusing to leave the house, or taking time off work due to stress).

The psychiatric system seeks to prevent risk-taking behaviour due to fears of suicide. This is understandable in some circumstances, but is misapplied "just in case" regardless of individual context. Recovery involves a balance of risk-taking with risk-aversion in a manner that is healthy for the person (Ramon et al., 2006, in Heller, 2015). This requires individuals to push themselves beyond their comfort zone without placing themselves in danger. Key to mental wellbeing is the ability to assess levels of risk appropriately and act on these findings with confidence. These aspects are considered in the following case study.

Case study: Godswill

St Mary's Hospital is a small psychiatric facility on the outskirts of a rural town in the north of England. It has facilities for adult and elderly people, and includes two admissions units and a rehabilitation unit. Through custom and practice the doors on the rehabilitation unit have changed from being occasionally locked at times of necessity, to being locked permanently. This situation contravenes guidelines on the Mental Health Act (1983), which encourages the least restrictive approach in patient care.

Godswill Ntini, a second year mental health nursing student, asks her mentor Natalie why the unit is locked. Godswill feels this practice is strange given the rehabilitative nature of the unit and best practice guidelines. In response, Natalie says: "Guidelines are fine in principle, but patient safety has to come first. There are patients on the unit detained under the Mental Health Act so we have to keep the door locked in case they escape. Otherwise it wouldn't be safe."

Godswill remains confused because there are a mixture of informal and detained patients on the unit. In her view, the principles of recovery are not being supported because staff fears for patient safety lead to the unit being automatically locked without regard for the negative impact this has on patients' self-esteem.

In this situation we witness contrasting interests between recovery-focused and traditional risk-averse mental health practice. Activity 7.2 asks the reader to consider this situation further, as it is not in the best interest of patients.

Activity 7.2   *Critical thinking*

Consider Godswill's case study. How might the risks described be better managed according to recovery principles?

A suggested answer is provided at the end of this chapter.

Godswill's situation, and the recovery-focused alternatives you have considered, illustrate contrasting approaches towards mental health patients. Natalie's viewpoint is based on an assumption that psychiatric symptoms indicate an inability for patients to make their own decisions. The discussion that follows demonstrates this is an unproductive approach to mental health work.

Recovery defined as the absence of symptoms

Achieving an absence of symptoms is sometimes referred to as "clinical recovery" (Petros et al., 2015). In practice, the achievement of this state is determined by mental health professionals, rather than patients (Macpherson et al., 2016). However, to regard recovery as merely the absence from the presence of symptoms is overly simplistic. This view is a misunderstanding of the causes of emotional and psychological instability, so is ineffective when planning mental health interventions. To accurately understand recovery, we need to consider the experiences of people in this process. Research studies report people in recovery as overcoming illness, and becoming well. Absence of symptoms do not necessarily occur for people in recovery, as the person may consider themselves recovered despite ongoing symptoms of varying degrees (Lariviere et al., 2015).

Recovery approaches have developed independently within both mental health and addictions sectors. Mental health and addiction issues are often artificially separated in practice through individual funding and service streams. In reality, overlap between substance use and psychosocial problems is significant. Relapse following periods of abstinence often occurs where underlying psychosocial and emotional issues remain untreated. Absence of psychological or addictive symptoms are not the target of recovery from substance use, but rather by-products of personal development to a healthier way of being. This process of personal development is worthy of further exploration.

Recovery defined as a voluntary process of personal development and wellbeing

Recovery from addiction is characterised by physical and psychological health that allows freedom of choice or abstinence from addictive behaviours (Kaskutas et al., 2015). If we adopt this approach towards mental illness, we reject a simplistic "ill" or "well" perspective towards our patients. Instead, symptoms of psychological distress represent an expression of their experiences, rather than indicating abnormality. By presenting symptoms as a normal reaction to extreme life events we avoid stigmatising our patients. Conversely, being labelled as mentally ill can be severely debilitating, becoming an aspect to be addressed during recovery.

The concept of wellness as a voluntary and active process is well recognised in theory. However, in practice a risk-averse system encourages service intervention "just in case" more than planning for long-term benefits. A lifestyle that focuses on maladaptive habitual behaviours, whether caused by addiction or symptoms of mental ill health, is often experienced as unfulfilling (Center for Substance Abuse Treatment, 2007, in Kaskutas et al., 2015). This perspective is not necessarily held by individuals using mental health services. Interventions attempting to enforce change under the Mental Health Act (1983) often disregard voluntary engagement as central to the recovery process, resulting in little positive change in the patient.

Recovery is a process of change from experiencing distressing symptoms, to emotional wellbeing. Through a highly personal experience of self-development, the recovering individual moves from a state of psychological instability, to regaining control over their life. This change occurs through learning to accept self-responsibility for their actions. Recovering from a period of severe mental ill health results in the individual undergoing a major review of their life, their attitude to self and others, and personal values. In order to achieve personal wellbeing, recovering individuals need to develop health-focused life skills (Anthony, 1993, in Tiderington, 2015). Recognising the possibility of independence in many aspects of life is key to achieving self-potential. The ability to self-manage our mental health improves as our experience of achieving self-determined change increases. The philosophy of recovery shares Carl Rogers' view of the fully functioning human being as synonymous with strong emotional health. Rogerian and recovery-focused approaches both promote the belief that it is only through ongoing personal growth that we can become content (Montellano, 2015; Rogers, 1961). Personal growth remains possible despite the presence of fluctuating psychiatric symptoms, emphasising the possibility of recovery progressing, despite emotional and psychological difficulties during the process (Petros et al., 2015). It is important that we do not underestimate the human ability to make life changes despite adversity, as people experiencing multiple co-morbid difficulties tend to respond better in recovery than those with less complex problems (Best and Aston, 2015). In these circumstances, continuous personal growth despite serious ongoing issues makes recovery even more significant for those undertaking it.

Severe psychological distress is one of the most feared and debilitating human experiences. It is therefore surprising that successfully recovered people often describe positive benefits from their experiences of emotional distress. Those who successfully undertake the in-depth examination of self required during recovery report being more attuned to themselves and others, and feeling more complete than before their emotional disturbance. Significant personal issues, rather than leading to upset, now become targets for future development (Noiseux et al., 2010, in Lariviere et al., 2015). Honest self-reflection is central to recovery, as through self-examination the individual recognises their unhealthy thinking and behaviour that contributed to their earlier self-destructive experiences.

Essential to dealing with personal problems is an honest appraisal of cause and effect. Future planning of this kind is necessary to determine what changes will be effective. Having recognised the unhealthy factors that created their distress, the person in recovery is better able to appreciate alternatives that will allow their functioning as a healthy human being. Many people who consider themselves to be successfully recovered achieve a healthy lifestyle directly opposed to their former way of being. Without things having gone wrong, they may not have developed such a healthy approach. The benefits felt through living well make life without distressing symptoms a realistic possibility once the person has developed their identity from sick to healthy individual. Recovery is therefore not a return to pre-illness norms, but the development of a state of being that is healthier than ever before (Best and Aston, 2015).

The role of the multi-disciplinary team in the recovery process

Recovery is a process of self-examination and individually determined action that impacts on every part of a person's life. The social aspects of personal wellbeing mean factors beyond the individual must be considered when developing recovery plans with service users. Where appropriate, the significant others of the person in recovery may have an important role in planning recovery. Unfortunately, their inclusion as equal members is often overlooked by multi-disciplinary teams in practice. This occurs because health professionals often fail to consider the wider social context of mental distress and recovery. The services and individuals most helpful in enabling recovery are housing organisations, criminal justice services and families.

Good quality, affordable housing is central to all aspects of health; therefore its provision is vital for successful recovery. However, knowledge of recovery processes is limited among personnel working in supportive housing and homelessness services (Gillis et al., 2010, in Tiderington, 2015). Service provision varies according to geographical location, with some areas inadequately resourced to provide specialist help needed for people recovering from severe mental distress. This is a false economy, putting pressure on mental health services to accommodate people who would otherwise be able to move from hospital to supported accommodation. Another significant factor is the disparity in quality of affordable housing available to people in recovery. In some areas, high housing costs make independent living without a sizable income unrealistic. This may seriously compromise recovery if people are forced to move away from existing support networks to find affordable accommodation, or are obliged to share living space with others they would not otherwise have chosen to live with. Housing costs remain a significant factor, disempowering people in recovery from becoming independent of services. Financial assistance may remain necessary to support living costs when people undergoing recovery do not have an adequate income. These factors illustrate the need to develop universal, well-funded strategic links between mental health and housing services, as well as a widespread knowledge of the recovery approach among professionals.

Contact with criminal justice services at various levels is a significant factor in the recovering population, in particular for those with a history of addiction. Patients who have received enforced treatment under the Mental Health Act (1983) may have undergone police interventions, sometimes on a number of occasions. Society's highest rates of mental illness are present within prison populations; therefore a recovery approach is critical within criminal justice services. However, collaborative working with mental health services remains uncommon in the criminal justice sector (Myers et al., 2016). UK prisons vary in their provision of mental health services, recovery-orientated approaches being the exception rather than the norm. The therapeutic community approach undertaken in HMP Grendon, Buckinghamshire, is an example of this.

Achieving social success may be a positive indicator of recovery (Macpherson et al., 2016). Social success contrasts with the perceived "loss of a normal life" commonly felt by patients experiencing severe mental health issues. Stable personal relationships are critical for the development of a self-concept strong enough to enable successful recovery (Leith, 2014). For these reasons, working with an extended social network rather than the patient alone is often beneficial in encouraging recovery.

For some people, their family and friends provide invaluable support during their recovery (Johnson, 2015). When crisis occurs, they may be able to act as intermediaries between services and service users. However, we have to recognise that complex family dynamics may have contributed to the development of psychological distress in the recovering person in the first place. Even when they are caring, families may not necessarily be the healthiest places to be when in recovery. Their lifestyle and values may no longer meet those of the person who is now in recovery, resulting in misunderstanding, conflict or encouragement to return to their pre-recovery way of being. Honest discussion between the patient and their family is critical in planning the early stages of their recovery. There may be outstanding issues or resentment between family members, so an honest appraisal of what is currently realistic for all parties when relating to each other is critical for the recovery process to proceed effectively.

Caring for someone who has psychological issues is emotionally demanding, often becoming a central factor in family life. Consequently, carers may need their own support. Rates of mental health issues are high in this group, and support offered by services may be insufficient for their needs (Johnson, 2015). Investment is required to support this group in the vital support they offer many patients undergoing recovery. Some families are reluctant to request help from mental health services because of a sense of shame about the issues experienced by their loved one. The role of the family varies between patients in recovery, but where successful provides an invaluable point of safety and stability. There is an opportunity for services to educate families on recovery principles, encouraging them to use these approaches themselves, and make challenging decisions rather than deferring them to professional services.

Rates of physical illness are much higher for people experiencing severe mental health issues than the general population. This is a consequence of stress and unhealthy lifestyle factors, commonly including consumption of multiple psychotropic medications. As a person recovers, their desire to live a healthy life develops to include physical as well as psychological factors. Poor physical health impacts on mental health, and good quality physical care services lead to better psychological outcomes (Leith, 2014). It is therefore unfortunate that physical healthcare has a minimal focus for many mental health professionals. Recovery-focused care requires the development of physical healthcare services that proactively meet the needs of people with severe mental health issues.

Obesity rates amongst psychiatric patients are extremely high due to poor diet, lack of exercise and the effects of medication (Brown et al., 2015). The negative impact of obesity on psychological health makes it an important issue to be addressed during recovery. When diet and exercise programmes are part of mental health treatment, participants are encouraged to take control of their appearance and physical wellbeing. The Nutrition and Exercise for Wellness and Recovery (NEW-R) curriculum is one example of a free, healthy lifestyle programme that has been positively evaluated by mental health service users, making it a highly suitable approach to implement in practice (Brown et al., 2015). Recognising areas for potential improvement within mental health services is important in developing best practice, as Activity 7.3 demonstrates.

Activity 7.3   *Team working*

Consider services relevant to people with mental health issues within your local area.

What aspects of the work provided by the NHS and third sector organisations are recovery-focused?

How could existing services develop to become more recovery-focused in future?

As this activity refers to your own practice area, an answer is not provided at the end of this chapter.

Having considered the realities of services relevant to your own practice area, it is now relevant to examine options when creating a recovery-focused service.

Operationalising recovery: techniques enabling recovery to take place

There is no single means of operationalising recovery (Andresen et al., 2003). Because recovery is unique in its scope and process for every individual, it is not straightforward to describe what a person must do to recover, or how care professionals can assist them achieving it. If services want to adopt a recovery-orientated system of care (Kaskutas et al., 2015), how can they do so if recovery can't be presented as a single defined process? One answer is for services to consider a range of approaches taken by people who have successfully recovered.

Recovery can take place individually, or as part of a group, depending on preference and resources available. Although not always necessary, undertaking therapy is often useful. The aspects addressed in therapy will depend on the aims and philosophy of the approach used. For example, if we consider the therapeutic approaches presented in Chapter 5, psychodynamic therapy may address healing from childhood trauma; CBT is useful in learning to control thoughts and emotions; person centred counselling enables self-acceptance; and brief solution-focused therapy can identify changes necessary in improving the person's life (Larivière et al., 2015, p. 560). Differences in approach highlight that the therapeutic approach chosen is less important than an ability to engage in change. If recovery is to become central to mental health work as many strategic policies claim, the workforce will need to develop psychotherapeutic skills to provide the range of support required.

As well as professional support for people in recovery, a critical role can be undertaken by peers who are also recovering from mental health issues. Support from members of the community is incredibly powerful in guiding and enabling positive self-development. Those who are successfully recovering are acutely aware of the difficulties experienced by others at earlier stages of the process, and the sense of hopelessness that can accompany the prospect of change. Sponsor or mentor roles may be used in addiction programmes, for example Alcoholics Anonymous and San Patrignano (see the case study on p. 147). Support from a successful, more experienced peer may be critical in encouraging people not to give up during early stages of recovery. This important responsibility highlights successful development of the sponsor, who is trusted to guide a highly vulnerable person at an earlier stage of their recovery. Despite recovery being a process that is highly personalised and focused on individual interpretation of meaning, it is nevertheless extremely useful to have the support, understanding and belief of other people in our ability to change (Russinova, 1999, in Myers et al., 2016).

Peer involvement in delivering recovery programmes demonstrates reciprocal relationships in action, giving purpose to those providing support. It inspires those in recovery by showing what a recovering person can achieve. Peers may be more convincing than professionals to inspire change. Early peer guidance in developing practical life skills may include joint development and monitoring of short-term and long-term goals, eventually occurring by the individual without practical peer assistance (Lariviere et al., 2015). The following case study examines recovery as a community-based process.

Case study: Recovery-orientated goals

Faith was diagnosed with a borderline personality disorder at eighteen. She experienced physically and emotionally abusive relationships as a young adult and spent time in prison for drug-related offences. Faith has made a number of suicide attempts, and has been cutting herself as a form of stress relief since her early teens.

After a number of years of brief and erratic contact with traditional mental health services, Faith began accessing a recovery-focused service for women diagnosed with borderline personality disorder.

During eighteen months of outpatient treatment, Faith was able to develop a greater contentment with life and a much healthier lifestyle. This was achieved through undertaking a recovery programme based on the following factors:

- *Ongoing participation in peer-led therapeutic group work based on self-acceptance and positive goal setting.*
- *Weekly individual cognitive behaviour therapy for six months.*
- *A course of **psychoeducation** on the impact of borderline personality disorder for the person experiencing it.*
- *Undertaking a life-skills training course – improving Faith's ability to cook, budget and care for herself.*
- *Improving her literacy skills through working with the educational specialist attached to the recovery programme.*
- *Participating in regular exercise, remaining drug and alcohol free, and reducing nicotine intake.*
- *Engaging in voluntary work and paid work placements with several local companies supporting the recovery programme.*

As a result of having undertaken this recovery-focused programme, Faith has remained living in her own home. She has not been arrested or sectioned under the Mental Health Act (1983) for three years.

Her mental health is much improved, she rarely self-harms and no longer plans to kill herself. She has learned to value her life without substance use, recognising its negative impact on her mood, thoughts and actions.

Faith has built a close network of healthy supporters, many of them in recovery, but also other friends from the wider community. She is much more physically active than she used to be, has a stable part-time job, and is at college studying maths and English. Faith has a goal to change her job for something that she finds more rewarding, but is unsure what this will be yet. She is not in a relationship but knows that feeling comfortable in being single is a massive positive change for her. Faith hopes to start a family one day.

Long-term planning and completion of life tasks of this sort are important for people who have lived fragmented and transient lives prior to recovery. In these situations little is permanent, therefore nothing substantial is completed. As well as goal setting, every day routines are a vital means of developing necessary life skills for independent healthy living. What many people regard as simple planning skills may be daunting for a person who lacked responsibility for their actions prior to beginning recovery. This is exaggerated further if they experienced **institutionalisation** through living in a penal or psychiatric system. Everyday tasks, such as maintaining appointments, cooking, cleaning, budgeting and paying bills, may be new or forgotten experiences for people recovering from periods of severe distress or addiction (Johnson, 2015; Lariviere et al., 2015). The need to achieve immediate practical tasks changes thinking patterns from negativity through dwelling on troubling past events, to a focus on current positive circumstances. This present focus allows the person in recovery to begin to let go of their past, instead focusing on life as it occurs for them. Witnessing personal success in routine practical tasks is an important part of recognising the self as a capable, independent being. The creation of a new identity based on competence and sociability replaces former identification with antisocial behaviour. Individual self-esteem is improved as group identity develops through communal activity. New members gain group membership through adopting and influencing the healthy behaviour and social values of other members (Best and Aston, 2015).

Case study: Recovery at San Patrignano Therapeutic Community, Italy

The role of companionship is central to recovery in therapeutic communities such as San Patrignano, where every aspect of members' lives involves community interaction, responsibility and support (Myers et al., 2016). Here, individual recovery is based on an expression of values present within existing members. The approach involves single sex work teams creating high quality products that are sold to enable the community to support itself. Participants describe their regaining of self-esteem and sense of belonging through a process of "contributing to society", "being productive", "getting

(continued)

continued . . .

something accomplished" and having "a reason for getting out of bed in the morning". Being immersed in a group that lives and works together provides a radically creative alternative to a pre-recovery life that was antisocial and non-productive. Programmes of practical and formal education are provided on site, from core skills to degree level study. Experienced group members guide new participants around their work and social systems; being surrounded by others creates conflicts that force partici-pants to develop skills to negotiate and resolve disputes in a healthy, non-aggressive and non-avoidant way. The community thrives through the respect held between members. Trust is developed through those guiding the community having themselves experienced extreme personal adversity in the form of addiction and mental health issues. San Patrignano claims a remarkable rate of recovery – around three quarters were maintaining a healthy lifestyle ten years after leaving the community.

The work undertaken at San Patrignano therapeutic community illustrates the development of individual autonomy through community integration. Autonomy is critical for success in recovery. It enables self-empowerment through accepting personal responsibility to develop necessary skills to survive independently in a healthy and sustainable way (Bledsoe et al., 2008; Liberman and Kopelowicz, 2002, in Myers et al., 2016). This involves replacing unhealthy, maladaptive coping mechanisms (such as drug use, anxiety or depressive symptoms) with flexible, realistic and healthy alternatives. For mental health service users to develop decision-making skills, decisions must be made jointly with them rather than for them by professionals (Adams and Drake, 2006, in Myers et al., 2016). Traditional mental health practice presents professionals in the role of guide to patients. Patients influenced by this type of practice may themselves prefer difficult decisions to be made for them. People who have experienced severe mental health issues, or who have long-standing addiction problems, may not be used to making lifestyle decisions because of the limited opportunities in their past life. A useful approach for mental health services is therefore to develop joint decision-making with patients based around everyday tasks of living (see Chapter 4). Once underway, this approach can build in complexity over time. Activities typically include self-care, cleaning of group areas and personal living accommodation, planning and cooking meals, shopping, seeking voluntary or paid employment, and undertaking informal or formal education. Less definable skills of social interaction are also critical for the person to develop a new sense of self no longer dominated by a viewpoint based on addiction or psychiatric symptoms.

Being supported in participating in social activities allows a person in recovery to re-engage in healthy interactions with other people. Social activities are a means of structuring time in a con-structive manner that ensures recovery does not become too internally focused. It also encourages physical activity and sociability, aspects that are often missing from pre-recovery lifestyles, but are vital for healthy development. Physical activity empowers participants to take personal responsi-bility for their own health. Regular exercise (often beginning with care of the physical environment) is a means of claiming back control of the body that was previously dominated by addiction or psychiatric symptoms. Exercise of any intensity is also a means of reducing anxiety and frustration. Cooperation in team sports allows bonding and expression of positive regard for other team members when directly verbalising these feelings may remain difficult. Critically, exercise of our own choosing is a means of expressing oneself and having fun without the use of substances or other maladaptive coping mechanisms, an aspect central to many accounts of successful recovery (Kaskutas, 2015).

A common theme reported by people in recovery is their search for a new personal identity. Previous troubling lifestyles dominate their identity until creation of a new one. Developing challenging personal interests is an important aspect of creating an identity beyond that of "person in recovery". Purposeful distractions from the recovery process are points of normality useful in recreating the self. The "meaningful day" concept highlights the need to set and achieve personal goals as a means of creating a new, useful self-identity. Here self-worth is enhanced through acting on constructive rather than destructive tendencies (Myers et al., 2016). Planning small and manageable changes leads to a larger process of planned achievement. This in turn enables the development of goal-setting skills that are useful in any future situation. In this way, planning and order replace chaos. The opportunity to experience a pattern of constructive activity during the early period of recovery provides hope and a precedent for future living. The replacement of inactivity and boredom with meaningful activity allows personal re-education to take place based around a healthy, socially constructive lifestyle and a genuine sense of purpose.

Volunteering and charitable activity are useful means of satisfying a reawakened urge to help other people that commonly occurs during recovery. This is a means of demonstrating personal social worth to wider society, and of making some redress for former antisocial activities. It benefits the person in recovery through their engagement in the demands of work, creating a record of vocational experience useful for potential employment, and a positive explanation of recent activity to potential future employers. The frustrating or boring aspects of voluntary work may also motivate the individual to seek more demanding employment. Pushing the self in a meaningful direction is critical to moving towards independence and away from needing professional support. This is the process of "letting go of the label of a mental illness to embrace life" necessary to create a new stronger identity than existed prior to recovery (Myers et al., 2016).

Abstinence is crucial in some recovery approaches, most famously the Minnesota model used by Alcoholics Anonymous, but may be less significant elsewhere. San Patrignano prohibits tobacco use in its programme, but has found success in a moderation approach towards alcohol, providing a small glass of wine at daily communal lunches and dinners. The responsibility to drink sensibly is placed with the individual, and those who wish to remain abstinent are supported in this by fellow members of the community. Non-problematic drug and alcohol use may not be achievable for many people in recovery, but is a realistic compromise for some, so should not necessarily be dismissed as an option. Non-usage of prescription drugs is recommended by some former mental health service users in recovery, directly opposing standard treatment from psychiatric services (Kaskutas et al., 2015).

Spiritual factors are often overlooked as important aspects of successful recovery. Spirituality may or may not include religious aspects, or a connection felt towards a higher power (this is central to recovery within the Minnesota model). Recovery may involve open-mindedness towards spiritual matters, and recognition of both individual insignificance and personal value within the world and wider universe. A practical means of expressing spiritual development may be found through assisting other people in their own recovery (Kaskutas et al., 2015).

Key to enabling successful recovery is the development of new social networks to replace former unhealthy relationships, and demonstrating an appreciation for existing supporters. Recovery relationships aim to be mutually supportive rather than imbalanced, with neither party being used inappropriately by the other (Kaskutas et al., 2015). New healthy relationships may fill emotional gaps felt by people who have poor family experiences, allowing them to move away from early painful experiences through choosing their own social contacts. Greater satisfaction with support networks developed during recovery indicates a higher chance of lasting positive change (Lariviere et al., 2015).

Self-reflection is necessary to understand and develop the personality within recovery. Engaging in psychotherapy is one means of guiding self-reflection in a positive and useful manner, allowing greater understanding of personal feelings and needs. Psychotherapy may be useful in recognising personal strengths and limitations, dealing with negative emotions and situations that previously caused significant distress. Self-reflection enhances our ability to deal with troubling emotions, instead making decisions that are influenced by logical, flexible thinking (Lariviere et al., 2015). As part of a group reflective process, Alcoholics Anonymous promotes those in recovery to consider what we personally can change and what we can't within any given situation. This is a means of preventing unnecessary distress, as factors beyond our control typically trigger the problem behaviours that dominated the person's life prior to their recovery (Kaskutas et al., 2015). Self-reflection is a key activity for success at every stage of recovery, the benefits of which are apparent through regular practice, as Activity 7.4 demonstrates.

Activity 7.4   *Personal development through self-reflection*

Recovery may be summarised as a process of identifying aspects of our lives that we need to change, and acting to enable these changes to take place.

Thinking about your own life:

- What significant changes have you made to your life since becoming an adult?

  o During the last ten years?
  o Since this time last year?

- What areas of your life do you recognise still need to change?
- What can you do to achieve necessary changes today, during the next week, next month, next year?

Because these answers are your own, a suggested answer is not available at the end of this chapter.

One thing that this reflective activity illustrates is that reflection is a process that can be applied to any aspect of our lives. Recovery shares this holistic nature, being an approach to living that can influence every aspect of our being.

As well as engaging in an individualised process of self-reflection, it is also possible to understand ourselves better through working with other people. Psychoeducation programmes may help participants to understand their personal mental health and the symptoms they experience. Psychoeducation is therefore a useful addition to individual and group therapy for those undergoing recovery (Lariviere et al., 2015). It may be delivered in a range of ways, but typically involves combined input from mental health workers and people themselves in recovery. This joint approach provides participants with professional expertise on technical matters relating to psychological and physical wellbeing, and role models who are successfully recovering despite experiencing similar difficult circumstances to their own (Best and Aston, 2015). Hope for personal change is consistently identified as vital in enabling successful recovery to take place (Lariviere et al., 2015). Structured support is often provided early in recovery programmes as a time of greatest need, with input reducing as the person gains independence (Macpherson et al., 2016). Peer recovery networks remain in use for many years by some people, others finding their own skills sufficient for permanent recovery to take place (Best and Aston, 2015).

It is clear from looking at recovery processes that significant differences exist between them and traditional, medically orientated psychiatric services. These differences in perspective are highlighted if we attempt to measure recovery. A medical approach measures patients' symptom severity, service use and hospital admission rates (Leith, 2014; Montellano, 2015). Successful recovery is determined according to patient and staff rating scales of patients' symptoms, disability and social function. These ratings typically diverge as patients feel they are recovering – that is to say, staff disagree with patients about the extent of their recovery (Macpherson et al., 2016). This supports the view that recovery is a highly personal experience and therefore impossible to measure objectively. As a lifelong process of self-development, a person cannot be said to have fully achieved recovery or failed to have recovered. Recovery is therefore a topic better suited to qualitative research, rather than quantitative measures that present recovery as an absolute success or failure.

The ultimate aim of a recovery-focused service is participant independence, no longer needing professional support to live a fulfilling life. Conversely, unnecessary engagement with services may restrict personal growth (Tiderington, 2015). Independence has to be the focus during any form of intervention. Unless it is shared by the patient, all professionals and significant others, progress towards recovery will be limited. A skills enhancing approach is therefore recommended to enable those in recovery to develop the skills to become fully independent.

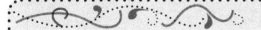

Chapter summary

Our exploration of recovery has considered both the philosophy underpinning it as an approach, and practical methods of its delivery. Recovery remains indefinable in any practical sense because it is a personalised process determined by individual needs. As human

(continued)

continued . . . . •

beings, these typically comprise of social, spiritual and health-focused goals for peaceful living. This lack of clear definition is understandable because to live someone else's values is never going to enable effective recovery. Discord between the individualised nature of recovery-focused approaches, and the restrictive, medically dominated psychiatric system make them fundamentally incompatible. If future services are serious about aspirations to provide more effective treatment for their patients, they need to be designed with a greater appreciation of evidence. The limited impact of medicalised psychiatry and the high suc-cess rates of pure recovery-focused systems such as the San Patrignano therapeutic community illustrate the need to redesign services. They must reflect what service users have found to work for them in achieving personal recovery, and what has hindered their progress. Such a change would represent a radical rethinking of mental health services and the loss of considerable professional power, with the views of current and former service users recognised instead as critical in determining what works for them.

Activities: brief outline answers

Activity 7.2 Critical thinking (page 140)

Where appropriate, patients' risk of self-harm due to absconding should be assessed on a daily basis. This allows the unit to be locked during times of high risk as a safety measure prior to transferring the patient to a more suitable secure setting.

To reduce risk of institutionalisation caused by being treated on the unit, patients should be encouraged to undertake healthy risk-taking activities through a therapeutic programme of visits into the local commu-nity, beginning with support from staff or relatives.

Re-education of staff may be necessary to promote positive risk-taking as a necessary aspect of recovery, and on the importance of using the "least restrictive alternative" prescribed by the Mental Health Act (1983).

Staff need to feel supported in their decision-making concerning risk – the multi-disciplinary team need to act in a united and evidence based fashion in its decision-making, and local policy needs to support positive risk-taking in the service.

Further reading

A detailed account of research on recovery and tools used to measure the process are provided in this document:

Campbell-Orde T, Chamberlin J, Carpenter J and Leff HS (2005) downloaded from **https://www.power2u. org/downloads/pn-55.pdf**

One of the more easily used recovery measurement tools is worth considering:

Tedeschi RG, Park SC and Calhoun LG (1996) Posttraumatic Growth Inventory (PTGI) available from: **http://www.emdrhap.org/content/wp-content/uploads/2014/07/VIII-B_Post-Traumatic-Growth-Inventory.pdf**

The STORI recovery scale is also very useful and available free of charge:

Andresen R, Caputi P and Oades L (2006) The Stages of Recovery Instrument: Development of a measure of recovery from serious mental illness. *Australian and New Zealand Journal of Psychiatry*, 40: 972–80. Available at: **http://socialsciences.uow.edu.au/iimh/stori/index.html#description**

Useful websites

The website of the Association of Mental Health Providers includes policy documents and practical resources relevant to recovery:

https://amhp.org.uk/

San Patrignano therapeutic community has an English language website including films featuring stories of people undergoing recovery:

http://www.sanpatrignano.org/en

Glossary

Abstinence: deliberate self-restraint from behaviours the person finds addictive – typically, the consumption of intoxicating substances such as drugs or alcohol.

Acute pulmonary insufficiency: a heart condition, where the pulmonary valve allows blood to flow in the wrong direction.

Agoraphobic: fear of enclosed spaces, or crowded places.

Arrhythmia: an abnormal heartbeat, including slow, rapid or irregular.

Attachment theory: theory suggesting early childhood experiences impact significantly on the way we think, feel and behave as adults.

Atypical: an aspect that is unrepresentative of the subject.

Bidirectional: factors that work in both directions.

Biochemistry: the chemical processes occurring within all living things.

Blood dyscrasias: an imbalance between plasma, white and red blood cells.

Cardiovascular: aspects relating to the heart and its blood vessels.

Catatonia: repetitive purposeless overactive movement, or conversely a lack of movement, rigidity and stupor in an individual.

Cerebellum: a section of the brain controlling movement.

Circadian rhythm disorders: issues with the person's internal body clock, affecting natural cues to sleep and wake up.

Coercive psychiatric environment: a mental health treatment environment that includes threat to individuals involved. For example, informal patients feeling they must take prescribed medication because they fear being sectioned under the Mental Health Act (1983) if they do not do so.

Cognitive: thinking patterns, usually in the form of inner verbal dialogue and images.

Cognitive impairment: limitations to the person's ability to think.

Co-morbid: the simultaneous presence of more than one disease or condition at the same time. Each condition may worsen the other.

Congruence: honesty of thoughts, feelings and behaviour, representing freedom from inner conflict.

Convulsions: involuntary severe shaking of the body caused by muscles rapidly contracting and relaxing.

Delusion: beliefs that are maintained despite evidence that is generally accepted as logical and rational.

Disorder: a state of confusion. In medical terms, this refers to differences from expected norms of physical or mental wellbeing.

Dopamine: a neurotransmitter acting as a chemical messenger in the brain.

Dysthymia: Persistent mild depression, representing fewer and milder symptoms than occur with more severe forms of depression.

Electro convulsive therapy (ECT): a psychiatric treatment that deliberately triggers small seizures in the brain through applying a small electrical current to the patient's brain. This is an attempt to make positive changes to brain chemistry.

Empowerment: the power or authority of a person or group to undertake specified tasks.

Euphoria: a state of happiness beyond reasonable expectations within a specific situation.

Evaluation: a judgement about the value of a thing or situation.

Family dynamics: individualised patterns of interaction between family members.

Gastro-intestinal issues: problems with the stomach or intestine.

Generic: something than is general or not specific.

Genitourinary: organs of the genital and urinary systems.

Grandiose: an unrealistic belief in personal self-importance, for example in terms of social standing or wealth.

Haemorrhage: heavy loss of blood from a burst blood vessel.

Hallucinations: perceiving the presence of things that are not really there. This could be an experience of any of the senses (sight, sound, smell, taste, touch).

Heartblock: a problem with the rate or rhythm of the heart.

Hierarchical nature: organisation of objects or people according to their perceived relative value compared to each other.

Histrionic: behaviour that is exaggerated beyond what would normally be expected in similar circumstances.

Holistic view: a consideration of the wellbeing of the whole person, rather than concentrating only on their state of health.

Hyperprolactinaemia: abnormally high prolactin levels in the blood.

Hypersalivation: excessive amounts of saliva in the mouth.

Hypersomnia: unusual and persistent sleepiness during the day, or excessive time spent sleeping.

Hyperventilation: an abnormally rapid rate of breathing.

Hypotension: abnormally low blood pressure.

Implementation: putting into effect plans or decisions.

Impotence: lack of ability of a man to achieve an erection, or to ejaculate.

Incongruence: disharmony occurring between thoughts, feeling and behaviour, often due to external influences. This can be described as a person not being themselves.

Insomnia: an inability to fall asleep or remain sleeping for sufficient amounts of time.

Institutionalisation: patterns of behaviour that follow institutional rules, persisting after the person leaves their institutional environment. For example, a person who has all of their meals provided for them during a long period of hospitalisation may lose the cooking skills they possessed prior to entering hospital.

Jaundice: abnormally high levels of bile in the blood, causing yellowing of the skin and eyes.

Learned helplessness: strongly held views of personal inability to make positive changes in life.

Lesions: damage to an organ of the body, including wounds, ulcers or sores.

Lethargic: feeling low in energy.

Libido: sexual desire.

Mental wellbeing: an individually determined state of mind represented not only by the absence of psychological disturbance, but also an ability to react realistically and effectively to difficulties experienced in life. Additionally, mental wellbeing is characterised by creativity and freedom of self-expression, rather than conforming to other people's expectations.

Mindfulness: conscious awareness of the present situation.

Mobilisation: making something ready for active usage.

Narcissism: excessive interest in oneself to the neglect of others.

Nausea: feeling sick.

Obstructive sleep apnea: repeated stopping and starting of breathing during sleep.

Ocular: aspects related to vision, or the eyes.

Oedema: swelling in an area of the body caused by build-up of fluid.

Osteoporosis: a disease that reduces quality and density of bones, making them more likely to break.

Palpitations: irregular, rapid heartbeat.

Paradoxical: a contradictory situation, where the opposite of what is naturally expected occurs.

Paraesthesia: feelings of "pins and needles" or burning without a physical cause.

Phobia: an irrational fear of a specific thing, persisting despite logical argument and evidence to the contrary.

Physiological: the healthy function of the human body.

Postural hypotension: blood pressure falling as a result of standing up.

Psychodynamic: theories of human psychology and interaction, originating from the work of Sigmund Freud, but further developed by subsequent psychologists.

Psychoeducation: a process of educating people, often in groups, about specific mental health conditions or approaches to mental wellbeing.

Psychomotor retardation: slowing of thought, emotional reactions, speech and physical movement in the individual.

Psychotherapy: any psychological form of treatment used to improve mental wellbeing.

Psychotropic medication: drugs marketed as improving mental wellbeing.

Punitive action: punishment as a direct result of specific actions or inactions.

QT interval prolongation: an abnormal extension of time between the heart's electrical cycles.

Re-acclimatise: to adapt to a situation or environment.

Recovery: the process of moving away from a life dominated by psychological and physical health issues, to one of greater harmony and purpose.

Respiratory: relating to breathing.

Risk-averse: reluctance by individuals or services to take necessary risks within patient care.

Schemas: strongly held beliefs that are used by an individual to organise and interpret information.

Sedation: becoming calm as a result of taking sedative medication.

Seizure: sudden abnormal electrical activity in the brain, resulting in convulsions.

Sleep apnoea: a disorder resulting in pauses, often repeatedly, of breathing during sleep.

Stigmatising views: regarding someone unfairly, particularly in terms of being less worthy than other people.

Stockpiling tablets: accumulating a large number of tablets, potentially as a means of overdosing.

Tachycardia: an abnormally rapid heartbeat.

Tinnitus: hearing noises, typically buzzing, whistling or ringing, that are not externally present.

Toxicity: poisoning of an organ, or the whole organism.

Traumatisation: psychological injury occurring through a shocking personal experience.

Vasodilation: widening of blood vessels.

References

Afonso P, Brissos S, Figueira ML and Paiva T (2011) Schizophrenia patients with predominantly positive symptoms have more disturbed sleep-wake cycles measured by actigraphy. *Psychiatry Research*, 189: 62–6.

Alfaro-Lefevre R (1995) *Critical Thinking in Nursing.* Philadelphia, PA: W.B. Saunders.

Alvarez-Jimenez M and González-Blanch C (2010) *Prevention of Antipsychotic-Induced Weight Gain in Young People with Psychosis: A Multi-Modal Psychological Intervention.* Santander, Spain: Publican-University of Cantabria Editions.

Alvaro PK, Roberts RM and Harris JK (2013) A systematic review assessing bidirectionality between sleep disturbances, anxiety, and depression. *SLEEP*, 36(7): 1059–68.

American Psychiatric Association (2013) *Diagnostic and Statistical Manual of Mental Disorders*, 5th edn. Arlington, VA: American Psychiatric Publishing.

Amital D, Fostick L, Silberman A, et al. (2013) Physical co-morbidity among treatment resistant vs. treatment responsive patients with major depressive disorder. *European Neuropsychopharmacology*, 23(8): 895–901.

Andresen R, Caputi P and Oades LG (2003) The experience of recovery from schizophrenia: Towards an empirically validated stage model. *Australian and New Zealand Journal of Psychiatry*, 37(5): 586–94.

Anita, S and Bhawna S (2015) Impact of medication, nutrition and routine exercise on mental health of patients. *The Bede Athenaeum*, 6(1): 216–19.

Anthony WA (1993) Recovery from mental illness: The guiding vision of the mental health service system in the 1990s. *Psychosocial Rehabilitation Journal*, 16(4): 11–23.

Barker P (2008) *Psychiatric and Mental Health Nursing: The Craft of Caring*, 2nd edn. London: Hodder Arnold.

Barrett D, Wilson B and Woolands A (2009) *Care Planning: A Guide for Nurses.* Essex: Pearson.

Beck AT (1973) *The Diagnosis and Management of Depression.* Philadelphia, PA: University of Pennsylvania Press.

Beck AT and Steer RA (1988) *Manual for the Beck Hopelessness Scale.* San Antonio, TX: Psychological Corporation.

Beck AT, Brown GK and Steer RA (1997) Psychometric characteristics of the Scale for Suicide Ideation with psychiatric outpatients. *Behaviour Research and Therapy*, 35(11): 1039–46.

Beck AT, Rush J, Shaw BF and Emery G (1979) *Cognitive Therapy for Depression.* New York: Guilford Press.

Beck AT, Schuyler D and Herman I (1974) Development of suicidal intent scales. In: Beck AT, Resnik HLP and Lettieri DJ (eds). *The Prediction of Suicide.* Bowie, MD: Charles Press.

Bental R (2003) *Madness Explained: Psychosis and Human Nature.* London: Penguin Books.

Best D and Aston E (2015) Long-term recovery from addiction: Criminal justice involvement and positive criminology? In: Ronel N and Segev D (eds). *Positive Criminology.* New York: Routledge/Taylor and Francis, pp. 177–93.

Black TR (2013) *Assessment of Suicide and Risk Inventory.* Available at: http://creativecommons.org/licenses/by-nc-nd/2.5/ca/

Bledsoe SE, Lukens E, Onken S, Bellamy JL and Cardillo-Geller L (2008) Mental illness, evidence-based practice, and recovery: Is there compatibility between service-user-identified recovery-facilitating and hindering factors and empirically supported interventions? *Best Practice in Mental Health*, 4(2): 34–58.

Bleich A, Baruch Y, Hirschmann S, Lubin G, Melamed Y, Zemishlany Z and Keplan Z (2011) Management of the suicidal patient in the era of defensive medicine: Focus on suicide risk assessment and boundaries of responsibility. *Israel Medical Association Journal*, 13: 653–6.

British National Formulary (BNF) 72. (2016) *September 2016–March 2017.* London: BMJ Group.

Brown C, Read H, Stanton M, Zeeb M, Jonikas JA and Cook JA (2015) A pilot study of the Nutrition and Exercise for Wellness and Recovery (NEW-R): A weight loss program for individuals with serious mental illnesses. *Psychiatric Rehabilitation Journal*, 38(4): 371–3.

Cade B and O'Hanlon B (1993) *A Brief Guide to Brief Therapy.* New York: Norton.

Centre for Addiction and Mental Health (CAMH) (2011) *Suicide Prevention and Assessment Handbook.* Canada: Centre for Addiction and Mental Health.

Christensen L (2001) The effect of food intake on mood. *Clinical Nutrition*, 20 (supplement 1): 161–6.

Coplan JD, Aaronson CJ, Panthangi V and Kim Y (2015) Treating comorbid anxiety and depression: Psychosocial and pharmacological approaches. *World Journal of Psychiatry*, 5(4): 366.

Corey G (2009) *Theory and Practice of Counselling and Psychotherapy*, 8th edn. Belmont, CA: Brooks/Cole.

Correll CU, Rummel-Kluge C, Corves C, Kane JM and Leucht S (2009) Antipsychotic combinations vs monotherapy in schizophrenia: A meta-analysis of randomized controlled trials. *Schizophrenia Bulletin*, 35(2): 443–57.

Cull JG and Gill WS (1988) *Suicide Probability Scale Manual.* Los Angeles: Western Psychological Services.

Cutcliffe JR and Barker P (2004) The Nurses' Global Assessment of Suicide Risk (NGASR): Developing a tool for clinical practice. *Journal of Psychiatric and Mental Health Nursing*, 11(4): 393–400.

De Moor MH, Boomsma DI, Stubbe JH, Willemsen G and de Geus EJ (2008) Testing causality in the association between regular exercise and symptoms of anxiety and depression. *Archives of General Psychiatry*, 65: 897–905.

Department of Health (1983) *Mental Health Act.* London: HMSO.

Department of Health (2005) *Mental Capacity Act.* London: HMSO.

Department of Health (2013) *The Francis Report: Report of the Mid Staffordshire NHS Foundation Trust Public Inquiry.* Mid Staffordshire NHS Foundation Trust. London: DOH.

Department of Health (2015) *Reference Guide to the Mental Health Act 1983.* Norwich: The Stationery Office.

de Shazer S (1998) *Clues: Investigating Solutions in Brief Therapy.* New York: WW Norton and Co.

Diamond A and Lee K (2011) Interventions shown to aid executive function development in children 4 to 12 years old. *Science*, 333: 959–64.

Dobson K (ed.) (2001) *Handbook of Cognitive-Behavioral Therapies.* New York: Guilford Press.

Dryden W and Yankura J (1993) *Counselling Individuals: A Rational-Emotive Handbook*, 2nd edn. London: Whurr.

Ellis A (1962) *Reason and Emotion in Psychotherapy.* New York: Lyle Stuart.

Evans G (2007) *Counselling Skills for Dummies.* Chichester: John Wiley.

Fiuza-Luces C, Garatachea N, Berger NA and Lucia A (2013) Exercise is the real polypill. *Physiology*, 28: 330–58.

Freeman D, Waite F, Startup H, et al. (2015) Efficacy of cognitive behavioural therapy for sleep improvement in patients with persistent delusions and hallucinations (BEST): A prospective, assessor-blind, randomised controlled pilot trial. *Lancet Psychiatry*, 2: 975–83.

Gorczynski P and Faulkner G (2010) Exercise therapy for schizophrenia. *Cochrane Database of Systematic Reviews*, Issue 5.

Hawgood J and De Leo D (2014) *Framework of a Suicide Risk Assessment Tool*. Australian Institute for Suicide Research and Prevention, Griffith University. Available at: https://www.psychology.org.au/Assets/Files/AISRAP%20protocol.pdf

Hawgood J and De Leo D (2015) *Screening Tool for Assessing Risk of Suicide (STARS)*. Australian Institute for Suicide Research and Prevention, Griffith University. Available at: https://www.griffith.edu.au/__data/assets/pdf_file/0004/625846/AISRAP-Suicide-Assess-Tool-2015.pdf

Heisel MJ and Flett GL (2006) The development and initial validation of the Geriatric Suicide Ideation Scale. *American Journal of Geriatric Psychiatry*, 14(9): 742–51.

Heller NR (2015) Risk, hope and recovery: Converging paradigms for mental health approaches with suicidal clients. *British Journal of Social Work*, 45(6): 1788–803.

Hermes B, Deakin K, Lee K and Robinson S (2009) Suicide risk assessment 6 steps to a better instrument. *Journal of Psychosocial Nursing*, 47(6): 44–9.

Hirdes JP, Marhaba M, Smith TF, et al. (2000) Development of the Resident Assessment Instrument – Mental Health (RAI-MH). *Hospital Quarterly*, 4(2): 44–51.

Hofstetter JR, Lysaker PH and Mayeda AR (2005) Quality of sleep in patients with schizophrenia is associated with quality of life and coping. *BMC Psychiatry*, 5: 13.

Holmes A, Murphy DL and Crawley JN (2003) Abnormal behavioral phenotypes of serotonin transporter knockout mice: Parrellels with human anxiety and depression. *Biological Psychiatry*, 54: 953–9.

Jansson-Frojmark M and Lindblom K (2008) A bidirectional relationship between anxiety and depression, and insomnia? A prospective study in the general population. *Journal of Psychosomatic Research*, 64: 443–9.

Johnson B (2015) Psychiatric rehabilitation. *Die Psychiatrie*, 12: 188–90.

Kaneita Y, Yokoyama E, Harano S, et al. (2009) Associations between sleep disturbance and mental health status: A longitudinal study of Japanese junior high school students. *Sleep Medicine*, 10: 780–6.

Kaskutas LA, Witbrodt J and Grella CE (2015) Recovery definitions: Do they change? *Drug and Alcohol Dependence*, 154: 85–92.

Kemp AH and Quintana DS (2013) The relationship between mental and physical health: Insights from the study of heart rate variability. *International Journal of Psychophysiology*, 89: 288–96.

Kiecolt-Glaser JK (2010) Stress, food, and inflammation: Psychoneuroimmunology and nutrition at the cutting edge. *Psychosomatic Medicine*, 72: 365–9.

Kourlaba G, Panagiotakos DB, Mihas K, Alevizos A, Marayiannis K, Mariolis A and Tountas Y (2009) Dietary patterns in relation to socio-economic and lifestyle characteristics among Greek adolescents: A multivariate analysis. *Public Health Nutrition*, 12: 1366–72.

Kutcher S and Chehil S (2007) *Suicide Risk Management: A Manual for Health Professionals*. Malden, MA: Blackwell Publishing.

Lai JS, Hiles S, Bisquera A, Hure AJ, McEvoy M and Attia J (2014) A systematic review and meta-analysis of dietary patterns and depression in community-dwelling adults. *American Journal of Clinical Nutrition*, 99(1): 181–97.

Laoutidis ZG and Mathiak K (2013) Antidepressants in the treatment of depression/depressive symptoms in cancer patients: A systematic review and meta-analysis. *BMC Psychiatry*, 13: 140.

Lariviere N, Couture E, Blackburn C, et al. (2015) Recovery, as experienced by women with borderline personality disorder. *Psychiatric Quarterly*, 86(4): 555–68.

Leith JE (2014) Recovery and transformations from loss in adults with serious mental illness. *Dissertation Abstracts International: Section B: The Sciences and Engineering*, 76(5-B(E)).

Liberman R and Kopelowicz A (2002) Recovery from schizophrenia: A challenge for the 21st century. *International Review of Psychiatry*, 14(4): 245–55.

Linehan MM (1981) *Suicidal Behaviors Questionnaire*. Unpublished inventory, University of Washington, Seattle, Washington.

Linehan MM, Goodstein JL, Nielsen SL and Chiles JA (1983) Reasons for staying alive when you are thinking of killing yourself: The Reasons for Living Inventory. *Journal of Consulting and Clinical Psychology*, 51: 276–86.

Lunsford-Avery JR, LeBourgeois MK, Gupta T and Mittal VA (2015) Actigraphic measured sleep disturbance predicts increased positive symptoms in adolescents at ultra high-risk for psychosis: A longitudinal study. *Schizophrenia Research*, 164: 15–20.

Macpherson R, Pesola F, Leamy M, Bird V, Le Boutillier C, Williams J and Slade M (2016) The relationship between clinical and recovery dimensions of outcome in mental health. *Schizophrenia Research*, 175(1): 14–27.

Maning J and Ridgeway N (2016) *The CBT Workbook of Anxiety*, 2nd edn. Suffolk, UK: West Suffolk CBT Service.

Markkula N, Harkanen T, Perala J, et al. (2012) Mortality in people with depressive, anxiety and alcohol use disorders in Finland. *British Journal of Psychiatry*, 200: 143–9.

McLeod J and McLeod J (2011) *Counselling Skills: A Practical Guide for Counsellors and Helping Professionals*. Maidenhead: Open University Press.

Michels F, Schilling C, Rausch F, et al. (2014) Nightmare frequency in schizophrenic patients, healthy relatives of schizophrenic patients, patients at high risk states for psychosis, and healthy controls. *International Journal of Dream Research*, 7: 9–13.

Miller DN (2011) *Child and Adolescent Suicidal Behaviour: School-Based Prevention, Assessment, and Intervention*. New York: Guilford Press.

Miller WR and Rollnick S (2002) *Motivational Interviewing: Preparing People for Change*, 2nd edn. New York: Guilford Press.

Miller W, Norman WH, Bishop SB and Dow MG (1986) The Modified Scale for Suicide Ideation: Reliability and validity. *Journal of Consulting and Clinical Psychology*, 54: 724–5.

Montellano P (2015) Why recovery is so important for affected people: Recovery – a collaborative journey with many companions. *Die Psychiatrie*, 12: 190–1.

Morphy H, Dunn KM, Lewis M, Boardman HF and Croft PR (2007) Epidemiology of insomnia: A longitudinal study in a UK population. *Sleep*, 30: 274–80.

Mulder R (2011) Problems with suicide risk assessment. *Australian and New Zealand Journal of Psychiatry*, 45: 605–7.

Myers NAL, Smith K, Pope A, Alolayan Y, Broussard B, Haynes N and Compton MT (2016) A mixed-methods study of the Recovery concept, "a meaningful day", in community mental health services for individuals with serious mental illnesses. *Community Mental Health Journal*, 52(7): 747–56.

Nakash O, Gerber Y, Goldbourt U, Benyamini Y and Drory Y (2013) Ethnicity and long-term prognosis after myocardial infarction: A population-based cohort study. *Medical Care*, 51: 137–43.

National Health and Medical Research Council (2013) *Australian Dietary Guidelines*. Canberra, Australia: NHMRC.

National Institute for Health and Care Excellence (2010) *The Treatment and Management of Depression in Adults (updated edition). National Clinical Practice Guideline 90*. London and Leicester: The British Psychological Society and The Royal College of Psychiatrists.

Neenan M and Dryden W (2004) *Cognitive Therapy: 100 Key Points and Techniques*. New York: Brunner-Routledge.

Nelson C, Johnston M and Shrivastava A (2010) Improving risk assessment with suicidal patients: A preliminary evaluation of the clinical utility of the Scale for Impact of Suicidality – Management, Assessment and Planning of Care (SIS-MAP). *Crisis*, 31: 231–7.

Nestler EJ and Carlezon WAJ (2006) The mesolimbic dopamine reward circuit in depression. *Biological Psychiatry*, 59: 1151–9.

Norman I and Ryrie I (2013) *The Art and Science of Mental Health Nursing*, 3rd edn. New York: Two Penn Plaza.

Osman A, Bagge CL, Gutierrez PM, Konick LC, Kopper BA and Barrios FX (2001) The Suicidal Behaviors Questionnaire-Revised (SBQ-R): Validation with clinical and nonclinical samples. *Assessment*, 8(4): 443–54.

Patterson WM, Dohn HH, Bird J and Patterson GA (1983) Evaluation of suicidal patients: The SAD PERSONS scale. *Psychosomatics*, 24(4): 343–5, 348–9.

Payne RA, Abel GA, Guthrie B and Mercer SW (2013) The effect of physical multimorbidity, mental health conditions and socioeconomic deprivation on unplanned admissions to hospital: A retrospective cohort study. *Canadian Medical Association Journal*, 185(5): E221–8.

Perlman CM, Neufeld E, Martin L, Goy M and Hirdes JP (2011) *Suicide Risk Assessment Inventory: A Resource Guide for Canadian Health Care Organizations*. Toronto, ON: Ontario Hospital Association and Canadian Patient Safety Institute.

Petros R, Solomon P, Linz S, DeCesaris M and Hanrahan NP (2015) Autovideography: The lived experience of Recovery for adults with serious mental illness. *Psychiatric Quarterly*, 1–10.

Posner K, Brent D, Lucas C, et al. (2008) *Columbia-Suicide Severity Rating Scale (C-SSRS)*. New York: The Research Foundation for Mental Hygiene, Inc.

Reynolds W (1987) *Suicide Ideation Questionnaire*. Odessa, FL: Psychological Assessment Resources.

Rogers CR (1957) The necessary and sufficient conditions for personality change. *Journal of Consulting Psychology*, 21: 95–103.

Rogers CR (1961) *On Becoming a Person: A Therapist's View of Psychotherapy*. London: Constable.

Roper N, Logan W and Tierney J (2000) *The Roper Logan Tierney Model of Nursing: Based on Activities of Living*. London: Churchill Livingstone.

Saha S, Chant D and McGrath J (2007) A systematic review of mortality in schizophrenia: Is the differential mortality gap worsening over time? *Archives of General Psychiatry*, 64: 1123–31.

Sallis RE (2009) Exercise is medicine and physicians need to prescribe it! *British Journal of Sports Medicine*, 43: 3–4.

Sanna L, Stuart AL, Pasco JA, et al. (2013) Physical comorbidities in men with mood and anxiety disorders: A population-based study. *BMC Medicine*, 11: 110.

Scarborough P, Nnoaham KE, Clarke D, Capewell S and Rayner M (2012) Modelling the impact of a healthy diet on cardiovascular disease and cancer mortality. *Journal of Epidemiology and Community Health*, 66: 420–6.

Simmons J and Griffiths R (2009) *CBT for Beginners*. London: SAGE.

Sjösten N and Kivelä SL (2006) The effects of physical exercise on depressive symptoms among the aged: A systematic review. *International Journal of Geriatric Psychiatry*, 21: 410–18.

Spoormaker VI and Van Den Bout J (2005) Depression and anxiety complaints: Relations with sleep disturbances. *European Psychiatry*, 20: 243–5.

Stange JP, Kleiman EM, Sylvia LG, Magalhães PVDS, Berk M, Nierenberg AA and Deckersbach T (2016) Specific mood symptoms confer risk for subsequent suicidal ideation in bipolar disorder with and without suicide attempt history: Multi-wave data from STEP-BD. *Depression and Anxiety*, 33(6): 464–72.

Tansella M, Thornicroft G and Lempp H (2014) Lessons from community mental health to drive implementation in health care systems for people with long-term conditions. *International Journal of Environmental Research in Public Health*, 11: 4714–28.

Taylor DJ, Lichstein KL, Durrence HH, Reidel BW and Bush AJ (2005) Epidemiology of insomnia, depression, and anxiety. *Sleep*, 28: 1457–64.

Thomas M and Drake M (2012) *Cognitive Behaviour Therapy Case Studies*. London: SAGE.

Tiderington E (2015) "We always think you're here permanently": The paradox of "permanent" housing and other barriers to recovery-oriented practice in supportive housing services. *Administration and Policy in Mental Health and Mental Health Services Research*, 1–12.

Whichelow MJ and Prevost AT (1996) Dietary patterns and their associations with demographic, lifestyle and health variables in a random sample of British adults. *British Journal of Nutrition*, 76: 17–30.

Williams S and Rajapakse T (2013) Physical illness and psychiatric comorbidity. *Sri Lanka Journal of Psychiatry*, 4(1): 22–4.

Wilson R and Branch R (2007) *Cognitive Behavioural Therapy Workbook for Dummies*. John Wiley: Chichester.

Wirt A and Collins CE (2009) Diet quality – what is it and does it matter? *Public Health Nutrition*, 12: 2473–92.

Wolff E, Gaudlitz K, von Lindenberger BL, Plag J, Heinz A and Ströhle A (2011) Exercise and physical activity in mental disorders. *European Archives of Psychiatry and Clinical Neuroscience*, 261: 186–91.

World Health Organization (1992) *The ICD-10 Classification of Mental and Behavioural Disorders: Clinical Descriptions and Diagnostic Guidelines*. Geneva: World Health Organization.

World Health Organization (2001) *Strengthening Mental Health Promotion*. Geneva: World Health Organization (Fact sheet, No. 220).

Wulff K and Joyce E (2011) Circadian rhythms and cognition in schizophrenia. *British Journal of Psychiatry*, 198: 250–2.

Wurtman RJ and Wurtman J (1989) Carbohydrates and depression. *Scientific American*, 260: 68–75.

Yildirim B and Özkahraman S (2011) Critical thinking in nursing process and education. *International Journal of Humanities and Social Science*, 1(13): 257–62.

Index